THE POCKET IDIOT'S GUIDE TO

The New Food Pyramids

by Elizabeth M. Ward, M.S., R.D.

ALPHA

A member of Penguin Group (USA) Inc.

ALPHA BOOKS

Published by the Penguin Group

Penguin Group (USA) Inc., 375 Hudson Street, New York, New York 10014, U.S.A.

Penguin Group (Canada), 10 Alcorn Avenue, Toronto, Ontario, Canada M4V 3B2 (a division of Pearson Penguin Canada Inc.)

Penguin Books Ltd, 80 Strand, London WC2R 0RL, England

Penguin Ireland, 25 St Stephen's Green, Dublin 2, Ireland (a division of Penguin Books Ltd)

Penguin Group (Australia), 250 Camberwell Road, Camberwell, Victoria 3124, Australia (a division of Pearson Australia Group Pty Ltd)

Penguin Books India Pvt Ltd, 11 Community Centre, Panchsheel Park, New Delhi—110 017, India

Penguin Group (NZ), cnr Airborne and Rosedale Roads, Albany, Auckland 1310, New Zealand (a division of Pearson New Zealand Ltd)

Penguin Books (South Africa) (Pty) Ltd, 24 Sturdee Avenue, Rosebank, Johannesburg 2196, South Africa

Penguin Books Ltd, Registered Offices: 80 Strand, London WC2R 0RL, England

Copyright © 2005 by Elizabeth M. Ward, M.S., R.D.

International Standard Book Number: 1-59257-492-0
Library of Congress Catalog Card Number: 2005932778

08 07 06 05   8 7 6 5 4 3 2 1

Interpretation of the printing code: The rightmost number of the first series of numbers is the year of the book's printing; the rightmost number of the second series of numbers is the number of the book's printing. For example, a printing code of 05–1 shows that the first printing occurred in 2005.

Printed in the United States of America

Note: This publication contains the opinions and ideas of its author. It is intended to provide helpful and informative material on the subject matter covered. It is sold with the understanding that the author and publisher are not engaged in rendering professional services in the book. If the reader requires personal assistance or advice, a competent professional should be consulted.

The author and publisher specifically disclaim any responsibility for any liability, loss, or risk, personal or otherwise, which is incurred as a consequence, directly or indirectly, of the use and application of any of the contents of this book.

Most Alpha books are available at special quantity discounts for bulk purchases for sales promotions, premiums, fund-raising, or educational use. Special books, or book excerpts, can also be created to fit specific needs.

For details, write: Special Markets, Alpha Books, 375 Hudson Street, New York, NY 10014.

This one is for my mother, Anne.

Contents

Introduction

Most people care more about what they put into their car than what they put into their body. It's no wonder: it's much harder to deal with feeding yourself. There's really no excuse for an unhealthy diet, however. Not with MyPyramid, the U.S. government's new icon for good nutrition. MyPyramid, which replaces the Food Guide Pyramid, provides 12 eating plans. One of the New Food Pyramid regimens is right for you.

What's to learn about better eating from MyPyramid? Plenty. Proper serving sizes, for starters (you'll be surprised!); how many servings of fruits and vegetables foster good health; how to eat on the run without blowing your diet; and how cheese and ice cream fit into a healthier way of eating.

You'll also discover MyPyramid's plan to help you move around more. Physical activity gets a thorough going-over in this book because it's part of determining your calorie needs, and it contributes to your well-being.

Sometimes, the simplest approach to healthy eating is the most effective. MyPyramid is a monument to personalization that's about as basic as it gets as far as eating advice goes. The best part is that the new food pyramids are useful throughout life even as your nutrient needs change.

As you read this book, you'll find morsels of information along the way to help you digest MyPyramid's dietary guidelines:

Pyramid Speak

Definitions of important terms.

Fun FAQs

Answers to frequently asked questions about eating and exercise.

Pitfalls

Warnings about what might derail your efforts to eat better and exercise more.

Power Point

Tips and tidbits to make healthy eating easier.

Acknowledgments

For such a solitary process, writing a book sure does involve a lot of people. Many thanks, once again, to my husband Tom and three daughters, Hannah, Hayley, and Emma. Not only did they put up with the long hours involved in producing another book, they supported me, in their usual style, every step of the way.

Trademarks

All terms mentioned in this book that are known to be or are suspected of being trademarks or service marks have been appropriately capitalized. Alpha Books and Penguin Group (USA) Inc. cannot attest to the accuracy of this information. Use of a term in this book should not be regarded as affecting the validity of any trademark or service mark.

A Blueprint for Healthy Eating

In This Chapter

- ◆ A new twist on an ancient icon
- ◆ MyPyramid gets personal
- ◆ The foundation of healthy eating
- ◆ Why slow and steady change is best

The great pyramids are unrivaled feats of engineering. Although no building on American soil even comes close to what the ancient Egyptians built, we have our own pyramid to brag about—MyPyramid.

So what if our pyramid is constructed from paper instead of stone and didn't take nearly as long to build? Our pyramid and theirs share some common ground. MyPyramid and the ancients' are carefully constructed monuments that harbor secrets. Like the great pyramids, there's more than meets the eye to MyPyramid.

Out with the Old

MyPyramid is not our first pyramid to promote good nutrition. It's the second icon with the same shape to come onto the nutrition scene in the last 13 years. You're probably familiar with the Food Guide Pyramid, released in 1992 by the United States Department of Agriculture (USDA). The Food Guide Pyramid was designed to help Americans over the age of two build a better diet.

The Food Guide Pyramid

In the Food Guide Pyramid scheme, grains occupied the pyramid's wide base. The Fruits and Vegetables groups, equal in size, sat atop the Grains group. As the pyramid narrowed, the next tier was equally divided by the Meat and Milk groups. Added fats and sugars were allotted the smallest space, just under the pyramid's apex.

The amount of space each food group occupied, as well as the number of recommended servings, was meant to convey the idea that a diet based on foods naturally rich in carbohydrates——grains, fruits, and vegetables——was the way to eat.

However, the Food Guide Pyramid was not intended to diminish the contribution of high-protein foods, such as milk, yogurt, cheese, meats, poultry, eggs, nuts, and legumes, by allotting them less room on the pyramid's face. The pyramid's design did suggest that you needed fewer servings of these foods for overall nutritional balance. The Food Guide

Pyramid advised minimal fats and oils and also discouraged sugary foods and added sweeteners that supply calories and precious few other nutrients.

MyPyramid

In 2005, the government retired the Food Guide Pyramid in favor of MyPyramid. What's better about MyPyramid? Plenty. For starters, MyPyramid promotes the latest nutritional science as reflected in the 2005 Dietary Guidelines for Americans. See the "A Rock Solid Foundation" section in this chapter for more on the Dietary Guidelines.

Power Point _____

> MyPyramid includes something the Food Guide Pyramid did not—physical activity recommendations. Why include physical activity in a plan largely devoted to a better diet? Because diet and exercise habits are inextricably linked when it comes to health.

The revised icon is also meant to jump-start consumer interest in eating right. That makes sense. Anything new that generates as much buzz as MyPyramid is bound to get your attention, but will you remain interested enough to continue using MyPyramid in the long run? Perhaps, especially because MyPyramid is no longer a one-size-fits all approach to building a better diet. Personalization is MyPyramid's crowning glory.

MyPyramid, And Yours

You can't tell by looking at it, but MyPyramid is not just one, but a dozen different eating plans. That's a far cry from the Food Guide Pyramid, which made it difficult to determine how many servings from each food group you needed every day, whether you are a 20-year-old male or 75-year-old female.

How will you know which of the 12 plans is right for you? That's the very purpose of this book. As you move from chapter to chapter, you learn about picking a pyramid plan that suits you, as well as exactly how to put the latest eating and physical activity suggestions into practice. Chapter 12 provides the details of putting together a daily eating plan, regardless of your recommended calorie level.

Let's Get Personal

Under the MyPyramid system, the amount of food you should eat from each of the food groups varies depending on your age, gender, and physical activity level. You may be wondering how each of these affects the number of recommended calories. Read on to find out.

Age

Remember when you were a teenager and you could eat until the cows came home without gaining weight? Now that you're in your thirties, forties, or fifties, every bite counts in the battle of the bulge. What gives?

As adults get older, their *resting metabolism*, the number of calories required to keep you going 24/7, slows down. The change in calorie-burning capacity begins in your mid-20s, when total body fat starts to slowly increase and lean tissue (mostly muscle) starts its decline.

Pyramid Speak

Resting metabolism refers to the number of calories your body burns to maintain basic functions, such as breathing.

Losing muscle drags down your ability to burn as many calories as you did when you were younger. That's because muscle tissue requires more calories to sustain itself than fat tissue. The more muscle you have on board, the greater your metabolic rate, 24 hours a day, 7 days a week, so you burn more calories even when fast asleep.

Generally speaking, the weight gain that happens with advancing age occurs because you continue to eat the same number of calories without maintaining or increasing muscle tissue through regular physical activity. You can easily notice a 5- or 10-pound weight gain in the course of a decade without eating more or exercising less. However, sedentary behaviors are highly likely to make weight gain worse as the years pass.

Children from age 2 to 18 are different from adults. Because they are still growing and developing muscle tissue, bone, and every other body parts, their caloric needs are higher on a pound-for-pound basis. Children need energy to fuel growth plus account for physical activity, unlike adults who are no longer in a growth phase.

Fun FAQs

Why do many women going through menopause gain weight in their abdominal area? Nobody knows for sure, but the decline in estrogen production in the ovaries is one potential cause of this type of weight gain. Lower estrogen levels diminish muscle tissue to the point of lowering resting metabolism, causing weight gain to concentrate around the midsection.

Gender

Sorry, ladies, most men burn more calories than women. Before the male-bashing begins, you need to consider that genetics is at fault. Men have more muscle, and women have more fat. It's as simple as that. Blame Mother Nature.

The difference in body composition between the sexes makes its mark early in life. Just before their teenage growth spurt is the time when boys' and girls' energy needs start to differ. That's why MyPyramid has set up different calorie levels for males and females beginning at age nine, as you will see in Chapter 3.

Does that mean you are bound by your genes? Nope. Women and men can increase or maintain their muscle mass by working out regularly. Incorporating some type of strength training two or three times a week is the best way to hold on to the muscle you have and to build new muscle tissue.

Physical Activity

It's a no-brainer: The more you move around, the more calories you burn, and the more you need to eat to maintain your current weight.

So if you're a reluctant exerciser, you may want to start giving some thought to how you will include more physical activity in your daily routine. Chapter 2 delves into the details of physical activity.

Anatomy of MyPyramid

As you can see from the picture on the cover of this book, MyPyramid is one colorful symbol. Sure, it's pretty, but what does it all mean? Good question. The color bands in MyPyramid represent three of its basic principles. The five food groups, as well as oils, are symbolized by bands that differ in color and width, suggesting a variety of foods is needed every day for good health.

Here's what each color stands for:

- ◆ Orange for grains
- ◆ Green for vegetables
- ◆ Red for fruits
- ◆ Yellow for oils
- ◆ Blue for milk
- ◆ Purple for meat and beans

The bands differ in width to convey proportionality. For example, the Orange band (grains) is wider than the Yellow band (oils), giving the impression that grains take preference over oils.

Moderation is represented by the way the bands narrow from the base of MyPyramid to its pinnacle. Within most of the food groups, there are choices that contain little or no naturally-occurring or added fat, such as lean meats, fat-free milk, and oatmeal, and choices that do, including salami and bologna, ice cream, and doughnuts. The idea is to pick foods from each of the food groups that fall at the wider area of the band——the base of the pyramid.

Nobody, including the government, expects you to overhaul your eating and exercise habits overnight. MyPyramid's tag line, *Steps to a Healthier You*, suggests you can benefit by taking small steps to improve your eating and lifestyle habits. The stick figure scaling the pyramid in the picture on the cover of the book reminds you of the importance of daily physical activity.

Pitfalls

The recommendations in the Dietary Guidelines are intended for healthy people over the age of two. MyPyramid is not a therapeutic diet for any specific health condition. Individuals with a chronic health condition should consult with a health-care provider to determine the dietary pattern most appropriate for them.

A Rock Solid Foundation

MyPyramid wasn't constructed out of thin air. The 2005 Dietary Guidelines for Americans, a joint effort of the United States Department of Agriculture and the U.S. Department of Health and Human Services, serve as the blueprint for MyPyramid's eating and physical activity advice.

The Dietary Guidelines for Americans provide suggestions for people two years of age and older about how proper dietary habits promote wellness while reducing the risk of major chronic diseases, including heart disease and cancer. They also include recommendations for daily physical activity.

Under the very best of circumstances—eating what you should and getting the suggested amount of physical activity nearly all the time——here's how your diet might improve by following a MyPyramid eating plan.

You would:

- Increase your intake of vitamins, minerals, dietary fiber, and other essential nutrients, especially those that are often low in typical American diets.

- Eat less saturated fat, trans fats, and cholesterol.

- Eat more fruits, vegetables, and whole grains to decrease the risk for some chronic diseases, such as diabetes, heart disease, and some cancers.

- Balance your caloric intake with your energy needs to head off extra weight or promote a healthy weight.

Wow. Those are some lofty goals, especially if your diet is way off the mark. Don't get discouraged! Nobody expects perfection, especially right from the beginning.

> **Fun FAQs**
>
> What is a healthy diet? The Dietary Guidelines describe a healthy diet as one that emphasizes fruits, vegetables, whole grains, and fat-free or low-fat milk and milk products. It includes lean meats, poultry, fish, beans, eggs, and nuts; and it's low in saturated fats, trans fats, cholesterol, salt (sodium), and added sugars.

Slow and Steady

When it comes to changing our lifestyles for the better, Americans want instant gratification. We expect quick results from self-imposed dietary deprivation, and we usually get them. But restrictive diets and excessive exercise regimens backfire because we miss our favorite foods and we come to hate working out; as a result, we rarely change our ways for good.

Gradually adopting a lifestyle that incorporates healthier eating and more physical activity is what most benefits your waistline and overall well-being. Whether you're trying to shed some pounds or struggling to maintain your weight, simple changes help fight an expanding waistline.

If you've ever been discouraged about changing your lifestyle for the better, you'll revel in MyPyramid's mantra, *Steps to a Healthier You.* The health experts who designed MyPyramid firmly believe Americans can dramatically improve their overall health by making small improvements to their diets and by incorporating regular physical activity into their daily lives.

Do This Every Day	See This Change After One Year
Burn 100 extra calories without changing your overall caloric intake	10-pound weight loss
Eat 100 fewer calories without changing overall physical activity	10-pound weight loss
Both of the above	20-pound weight loss

It may be difficult to imagine that you could reap tremendous benefits from slight adjustments in your eating and physical activity routines. As long as you stick with small improvements, and you are willing to wait, you will be duly rewarded.

No Pyramid Is Perfect

Let's face it. No matter how hard you try, you can't please everyone, especially if they are health experts who make it their business to communicate how people can change for the better. Although

MyPyramid's architects get kudos for devising a system that personalizes dietary recommendations and promotes regular physical activity, the symbol itself leaves a lot to be desired.

It's unfortunate that a picture of MyPyramid cannot stand alone and be readily understood. That's one thing the Food Guide Pyramid had going for it: a quick glance conveyed the importance of basing your diet on plant foods while providing a range of servings from the other food groups. The current incarnation of pyramid as eating tool takes a lot of explaining. Which is why you're reading this book.

But never mind! As it turns out, you don't have to be concerned with the pitfalls of MyPyramid because this book has already found every which way around them for you. All you have to do now is proceed to Chapter 2 to take steps toward choosing the pyramid plan that best suits you. What are you waiting for? Get a move on!

The Least You Need to Know

♦ MyPyramid is actually 12 different pyramids.

♦ Caloric needs are based on age, gender, and physical activity.

♦ MyPyramid is derived from the 2005 Dietary Guidelines for Americans.

♦ Small lifestyle changes, over the course of time, add up to better health.

Figuring Physical Activity

In This Chapter

- The benefits of physical activity
- How much physical activity you need
- Your target heart rate
- Rate your physical activity level
- Ways to work in daily exercise

What is physical activity? If you have to ask, you probably don't get much. There's good news for confirmed couch potatoes and avid exercisers alike. Physical activity is not confined to sweating at the gym in Spandex workout gear; mowing the lawn counts toward MyPyramid's recommended daily activity quotas, too.

Because you already know your age and gender, you need one last piece of information before choosing a MyPyramid eating plan that's right for you. This chapter helps you assess your physical activity level; shows you why it pays to move around; and provides activity tips for even the most reluctant exerciser.

Why You Need Physical Activity

It's simple. Your body was designed to move. Physical activity, whether it's walking, gardening, or rollerblading, plays a major role in living a longer life that's relatively free of chronic conditions that sap your energy and take the joy out of living.

Go on, admit it: You feel better after you exercise. Even if you don't like how physical activity makes you feel while you're doing it, you definitely reap major benefits by being active. Regular physical activity:

- Burns calories and aids weight management
- Promotes self-esteem
- Reduces depression and anxiety
- Lowers your risk of colon cancer
- Strengthens muscles
- Reduces your risk for developing type 2 diabetes and promotes better management of blood glucose levels in type 1 and type 2 diabetes
- Lowers the levels of total and LDL (low-density lipoproteins) or "bad" cholesterol and higher concentrations of HDL (high-density lipoproteins) or "good" cholesterol in the blood
- Strengthens your heart and lowers your pulse rate
- Promotes a healthy blood pressure

- Reduces stress
- Builds stronger bones
- Makes for more limber joints
- Improves your circulation
- Sharpens mental acuity

Power Point _____

Exercise may head off breast cancer in women. Preliminary evidence suggests that premenopausal women who exercise moderately for three hours a week lower their breast cancer risk by 30 percent; women who work out four or more hours weekly were 50 percent less likely to develop breast cancer.

Hopefully, you found at least one benefit of physical activity to pique your interest in making it a part of your life ... which begs the question of quantity.

How Much Exercise Is Enough?

Any physical activity is good, but adults require a certain amount of movement every day. How much depends on what you're after in terms of weight control and health.

If you want to reap some health benefits and maintain your weight, 30 minutes each day of physical activity is enough. For health benefits plus preventing weight gain, MyPyramid says to shoot for at least

60 minutes. You'll need between 60 and 90 minutes of physical activity daily for maintaining weight loss while benefiting from a health standpoint.

The recommendations are different if you're under age 18. According to MyPyramid, children and teenagers should be physically active for at least 60 minutes on most days of the week.

Fun FAQs

How much exercise should pregnant women get? The 2005 Dietary Guidelines for Americans say that if your pregnancy is without medical complications that prohibit exercise, you should get 30 minutes a day of moderate-intensity exercise. Sorry, no horseback riding, skydiving, or skateboarding for the next few months! These activities are too dangerous. Ask your doctor about how much physical activity and what kind is best for you when you're expecting.

Some Activities Are Better Than Others

You're clear on the fact that you need at least a half hour of daily physical activity. Cleaning the house or getting up from your desk dozens of times certainly qualifies as activity. Yet it's not exactly what the architects of MyPyramid had in mind when they issued their exercise edicts.

MyPyramid's suggested level of physical activity is in addition to your usual activity. Sure, when you're sedentary, any activity is better than none. Taking a few five-minute walks during your day, or even raking the yard when you did not before, means you are taking small steps toward including the minimum amount of physical activity to stay healthy.

Not all movement counts toward better health, however. Getting up from your recliner to change the channel on the TV consumes more energy than using the remote control, and, when combined with other small activities, may even help with weight control. But that type of low-level movement won't strengthen your cardiovascular health, reduce your risk for certain cancers, or benefit wellness in any other way. For that, you need more strenuous exercise.

Moderate Physical Activity

Moderate physical activity is anything that boosts your heart rate to between 60 to 73 percent of its peak. (See the following "Target Heart Rate" section for more information.)

Although moderate physical exercise is challenging, you should be capable of carrying on a conversation comfortably while working out. Of course, that may look silly when you're talking to yourself at the gym or walking alone in the park. But you get the idea. Here are some examples of activities that could qualify as being moderate in intensity:

- Brisk walking (about 3½ miles per hour)
- Hiking
- Gardening/yard work
- Dancing
- Golf (walking and carrying clubs)
- Biking (less than 10 miles per hour)
- Weight training (general light workout)

Vigorous Physical Activity

Any activity that elevates your heart rate to between 74 and 88 percent of your peak heart rate is considered vigorous. It doesn't take a genius to figure out that vigorous exercise is more intense than moderate. The reason: it provides much more of a challenge to your heart and lungs. Vigorous physical activities include:

- Mowing the lawn with a nonmotorized push mower
- Running/jogging (5 miles per hour)
- Biking (more than 10 miles per hour)
- Swimming (continuous freestyle laps)
- High-impact aerobics
- Walking very fast (4½ miles per hour)
- Heavy yard work, such as chopping wood
- Weight lifting (vigorous effort)
- Basketball (competitive)

Pitfalls

Most people can add low-level physical activity, such as walking, without health repercussions. However, if you have a medical condition, including diabetes, heart disease, high blood pressure, asthma, or osteoporosis; or if you're over age 40, a smoker, very overweight, or you haven't exercised in years, check with your physician first for physical activity recommendations.

Target Heart Rate

What seems like a vigorous activity to one person is a piece of cake for the next. That's where working out within your target heart zone comes into play. Knowing your target heart rate (another word for pulse) is the first step toward figuring out your target heart zone, which allows you to measure your initial fitness level and monitor your progress.

Take Aim

Target heart rate is based on age. It's a useful guideline for measuring exertion, especially when you're just starting an exercise program.

According to the American Heart Association, you should aim for working out at 50 percent of your target heart rate during the first few weeks of exercise, and gradually build up. If you're already in shape, you may be capable of working out at upwards of 85 percent of your maximum heart rate. That's because your heart is strong so it doesn't need to work as hard to pump blood out to your extremities.

Use the following equation to calculate your target heart rate. You may need a calculator:

1. 220 – your age (in years) = target heart rate (beats per minute)

2. Answer from #1 × .60 = lower end of target for moderate physical exercise.

3. Answer from #1 × .74 = upper end of target for moderate physical exercise

Example: 43-year-old

1. 220 – 43 = 177 beats per minute

2. 177 × .60 = 106.2

3. 177 × .74 = 130.9

4. Exercise within this zone: 106 to 131 beats per minute

Are You in the Zone?

You know how many times a minute your heart should beat during moderate or vigorous exercise. Now measure it by taking your pulse. There are two ways to measure pulse; a watch or clock is required for both.

To take your pulse at your neck, place your index and middle fingers in the groove on either side of your esophagus, the hard pipe in the middle. Gently press against this artery. You'll feel a steady pounding of blood. Count the number of beats you feel in a 15-second block and multiply that number by four to get beats per minute.

To use the wrist method, place the tips of your middle and index fingers on the opposite wrist, just below the base of your thumb. After you find a steady rhythm, start counting. Proceed as if you were taking a neck pulse.

For fuss-free heart rate readings, consider purchasing a heart rate monitor. Heart rate monitors track exertion based on heart rate throughout your entire exercise session.

It's a good idea to take your pulse halfway through an exercise session. The idea is to pace yourself to reap the greatest health benefits. Measuring your heart rate at the beginning of a workout may give you the idea that you're not working hard enough when in fact you are just warming up; taking your pulse right at the end may not accurately portray how hard you worked throughout.

 Power Point _____

Certain medications used to treat high blood pressure also lower your maximum heart rate, which in turn reduces target heart rate. Ask your physician if any of the medications you take has this effect and how to adjust your target heart rate to account for it.

How Active Are You?

Many adults confuse mental fatigue with physical exhaustion. What's the problem with that? They think they are far more physically active than they actually are—because they are tired—which leads to overestimating caloric need. Eating more calories than you burn is a recipe for weight gain.

Before you use a MyPyramid plan to improve your eating habits, you must first assess your activity level in order to balance calories coming in from food and beverages and the calories you burn. Read on to figure out which activity category you fall into.

Sedentary

You get about 10 minutes of walking in while on your way to and from work, or when shuttling the kids to and from school. You may clean the house or mow the lawn or do some other concentrated amount of activity every other day or so. Or you go to the gym or jump on your home treadmill or stationary bike and work out for about half an hour every other day. You may feel like you never sit down, but by MyPyramid's standards, you're sedentary.

In pyramid-speak, sedentary means your lifestyle is pretty much devoid of physical activity during your leisure time. You get less than 30 minutes of physical activity every day.

Sedentary folks have a few choices:

- ◆ To keep your weight where it is without adding any physical activity, choose a pyramid eating plan with the least amount of calories for your age and gender. You'll maintain your weight, but you won't do your health any other favors.

- ◆ To lose weight, choose the least amount of calories for your age and gender and gradually increase your physical activity level to at least 30 minutes a day.

- ◆ If you'd like to eat more and maintain your weight, choose a level of calories between the highest and lowest for your age and gender, and gradually increase physical activity to 30 minutes a day.

Moderately Active

You bike to and from work, for a total of about 40 minutes every day. Or, you're the type of person who walks on his lunch break, working in a 40-minute workout five days a week. On weekends, you make it to the gym to ride the stationary bike, or take an hour-long, low-impact aerobics class.

Your activity level qualifies as moderately active, which MyPyramid defines as getting 30 to 60 minutes of physical activity daily. As long as your weight is within a healthy range, choose the calories under Moderately Active in Chapter 3 for weight maintenance.

Active

You're up with the birds to get that 60-minute run in before work or before you start your day at home. Maybe you use your exercise time to attend hour-long kickboxing aerobic classes at your local gym after work three times a week, taking an hour-long walk on the off-days. You get around!

Your activity level ranks as active, taking up between 60 and 90 minutes every day. As long as you're at a healthy weight that you want to maintain, choose the calories under the Active heading for your age and gender. And keep up the good work.

About Strength Training

By and large, MyPyramid's suggested activities to provide health benefits and burn the most calories qualify as *aerobic* activities that employ the large muscle groups, like those located in the legs and arms. When done long enough and hard enough, aerobic activities, such as walking and biking, challenge your heart and lungs, requiring large amounts of oxygen from the air you breathe. Taken literally, aerobic means "with air."

According to MyPyramid, light strength training falls under the heading of moderate physical activity; applying more vigor categorizes strength training as vigorous. This is somewhat confusing because it's hard to imagine sustaining an activity such as weight training for 30 minutes. Weight

training is an *anaerobic* exercise, a stop-and-go
activity that works on one muscle group at a time
and cannot be sustained for more than a minute or
two.

Pyramid Speak

Aerobic means "with air." Aerobic activities are repetitive and require oxygen from the air you breathe. **Anaerobic exercise** exhausts smaller muscle groups and does not require as much oxygen because the demand on the heart and lungs is not sustained.

That's not to discount strength training, which is
an important part of any physical activity regimen.
Activities such as weight lifting, weight machines,
and resistant band workouts strengthen muscles.
Strength training improves posture, tones your
body, strengthens bones, increases lean body mass,
and burns calories. Make room in your exercise
schedule for strength-training activities two or
three times a week.

Get a Move On

Moving around and working out has so much to
offer, and you want to be more active, but how?
You don't have the time or money to join a gym, or

maybe that's just not your scene. And you can't imagine lacing up your sneakers for a vigorous 30-minute walk during your busy day, especially when you barely have time to eat lunch while working at your desk. As luck would have it, there are ways around a lack of time or motivation or any other reason you can come up with to sit on your duff.

Pitfalls

Video, television, and computer screens around the house are stiff competition for physical activity, especially when it comes to kids. The American Academy of Pediatrics recommends less than two hours a day of "screen time" for children over the age of two. Allowing televisions and computers in a child's bedroom sets the tone for inactivity at a time when childhood obesity rates are at an all-time high.

Keep It Interesting

There's nothing like boredom to kill the motivation to move around more. Choose an activity, or two, that you enjoy and alternate them. Enlist an exercise buddy or join a walking group in the neighborhood or at the local mall; taking an exercise class is a good way to get motivated by others, too. Try a new activity to get motivated, such as spinning or dance class; yoga, pilates, or T'ai Chi. Listening to music or watching your favorite TV program or a movie while walking on the treadmill or riding a stationary bike at home are ways to multitask while working out.

Break It Down

Yes, your body needs a minimum of 30 minutes of daily physical activity. If that's daunting, there's good news. Even the most time-crunched people can reap health benefits with as little as three 10-minute bouts of physical activity throughout the day.

Making physical activity a part of your regular routine can help you stay active on most days of the week. You're ready to roll on a moment's notice when you keep a pair of walking or running shoes at the office or in the car.

Power Point

Schedule exercise time on your calendar and treat it as any other important appointment. No matter what activity you choose, plan your workouts and keep a log of your physical activity to boost motivation.

Here are some ways to work in 10 minutes of physical activity:

♦ Park your car farther away from your workplace and walk for 10 minutes to and from work. Get out for another 10-minute block of time during the day, and you're done.

- Bike to work.
- Walk the dog instead of letting him out the back door.
- Pedal an exercise bike or jump on a treadmill.
- Replace a coffee break with a brisk 10-minute walk. Ask a friend to go with you.
- Walk while waiting for the plane at the airport.
- When traveling for work or pleasure, stay at hotels with fitness centers or swimming pools and take advantage of the chance to be active.
- Pack a jump rope in your suitcase when you travel. Jump and do calisthenics in your hotel room.
- Put on your favorite music and dance around your living room.

Work Out at Home

Many people prefer to exercise at home; they find working out at home is more convenient, more private, or both. You may swear by your home treadmill or stationary bike. More power to you. But don't feel you must invest in expensive equipment to work out at home; chances are, it will just end up collecting dust anyway.

Exercise videos can help satisfy an urge to be more active right in your own living room, but make sure they are the right strategy for you. Home exercise videos are often like TV cooking shows—more fun to watch than imitate. Choose the risk-free route of exercising to a free workout show on cable television stations that last between 30 and 60 minutes. Or you may be able to check out an exercise video from your local library

Hiking, biking, and swimming close to home are other ways of working out that can involve the entire family. With the elimination of recess and gym from many schools, it's important for parents to encourage children to get their daily activity.

The Least You Need to Know

- You need a minimum of 30 minutes of daily physical activity.
- MyPyramid's recommendations are in addition to normal physical activity.
- Moderate and vigorous exercises offer the most health benefits.
- Make physical activity a part of your day by scheduling it in.

Chapter 3

Counting Calories

In This Chapter

- ◆ Discover your calorie quota
- ◆ Learn how to lose weight
- ◆ Combat portion distortion
- ◆ Spend your discretionary calories
- ◆ Find out what to feed children

Until now, you've barely given your diet a passing thought. Or maybe you've tried nearly every diet on the planet. Regardless, you're ready to eat right, once and for all, and you're eager to discover the blueprints for better eating. This chapter guides you to finding the MyPyramid plan that's best for you, and your child.

Consider Calories

Before you choose from the pyramid plans in Chapter 11, you'll need to determine how many calories are right for you to eat every day. Calorie levels for each of the twelve MyPyramid eating scenarios are based on age, gender, and your level of daily physical activity (which you have already determined from reading Chapter 2).

What does your calorie quota mean? It's the number of calories you need to consume to keep your weight right where it is at your current age and level of physical activity.

The charts that follow provide the number of calories recommended to maintain an adult's weight and to foster healthy growth in children. There are separate calorie levels for males and females starting at age nine, when males begin to need more energy from food than females.

Age	Sedentary	Moderately Active	Active
Boys and Girls, Ages 2–8			
2	1,000	1,000	1,000
3	1,000	1,400	1,400
4–5	1,200	1,400	1,600
6–7	1,400	1,600	1,800
8	1,400	1,600	2,000
Boys, Ages 9–18			
9	1,600	1,800	2,000
10	1,600	1,800	2,200
11	1,800	2,000	2,200
12	1,800	2,200	2,400
13	2,000	2,200	2,600
14	2,000	2,400	2,800
15	2,200	2,600	3,000
16–18	2,400	2,800	3,200

Girls, Ages 9–18			
9	1,400	1,600	1,800
10	1,400	1,800	2,000
11	1,600	1,800	2,000
12–13	1,600	2,000	2,200
14–18	1,800	2,000	2,400
Men, Ages 19 and older			
19–20	2,600	2,800	3,000
21–35	2,400	2,800	3,000
36–40	2,400	2,600	2,800
41–55	2,200	2,600	2,800
56–60	2,200	2,400	2,600
61 +	2,000	2,400	2,600
Women, Ages 19 and older			
19–20	2,000	2,200	2,400
21–25	2,000	2,200	2,400
26–30	1,800	2,000	2,400
31–50	1,800	2,000	2,200
51–60	1,600	1,800	2,200
61 +	1,600	1,800	2,000

Sedentary means less than 30 minutes a day of moderate physical activity in addition to daily activities.

Moderately active means at least 30 minutes and up to 60 minutes a day of moderate physical activity in addition to daily activities.

Active means 60 or more minutes a day of moderate physical activity in addition to daily activities.

Source:www.mypyramid.gov.

Bear in mind that although these charts consider age, gender, and activity, they serve as guidelines only. You may need to tailor these suggested calorie intakes to better suit your needs, decreasing or increasing calories as you see fit.

Weighing In on Weight

You may be happy with your weight, but would your doctor or dietitian be as thrilled? Find out by calculating your *Body Mass Index* (BMI) to be sure your weight falls within a healthy range. BMI relates your weight to your height.

 Pyramid Speak

Body Mass Index is a comparison of your height to your body weight. For most people, it's a reliable indicator of extra body fat.

Health professionals consider BMI a reliable indicator of extra body fat. However, BMI overestimates body fat for very muscular people. Not to worry, most of us don't fall into that category.

Here's how to figure your BMI. You'll need a reliable scale and, unless you're a math whiz, a calculator:

1. Weigh yourself naked first thing in the morning.

2. Multiply your weight in pounds by 700.

3. Divide the result in #2 by your height in inches.

4. Divide the result in #3 by your height in inches again.

That's your BMI.

Here's an example of how the BMI calculation works for a 140-pound person who is 5'6" tall (66 inches).

700 × 140 = 98,000

98,000/66 = 1484

1484/66 = 22.4

BMI = 22.4

A BMI under 19 means you may not weigh enough; a BMI between 19 and 25 means you're within normal range; and a BMI of 26 and above means you may need to shed some weight.

Maintaining Your Weight

Your BMI is within normal range. That is good news. Here's the not-so-happy part: Even when weight maintenance is your goal, chances are you'll need to eat less every year, so keep making the necessary calorie adjustments with each birthday.

A moderately active 25-year-old female requires about 2,200 calories a day to keep her weight stable. That same woman should be consuming 400 fewer calories by age 51, unless she has dramatically increased her physical activity level. Why? Because time robs the body of lean tissue. Lean tissue (muscle, mostly) burns more calories than fat tissue, so calorie-burning capacity declines as you get on in years.

When you continue eating the same number of calories without maintaining or increasing muscle mass through exercise, you'll probably gain weight. Does that mean you must become big and bulky to burn calories? Not at all, but it does mean you'll probably need to add weight training to your exercise regimen to retain the muscle you have.

Pitfalls

People who must lose weight to help manage or prevent a chronic condition, such as diabetes or heart disease, can use a MyPyramid eating plan. However, it's best to consult with a registered dietitian (R.D.) first. An R.D. is able to coordinate your diet, physical activity, and any medications you take on a regular basis.

What to Do for Weight Loss

Your BMI is too high. The good news is that MyPyramid provides a sound foundation for losing weight and keeping it off with a balanced diet and regular physical activity.

Here's how to get started on losing weight by eating less. Determine the number of calories you need to maintain your current weight, which you have already accomplished by consulting the tables provided at the beginning of this chapter.

From there, subtract 500 calories from your daily calorie quota to lose about one pound a week.

Here's why that approach works for most people. A pound of body fat contains 3,500 calories. Over the course of seven days, you need to decrease food intake by a total of 3,500 calories, which amounts to a daily deficit of 500.

Although adults might like to carve out more than 500 calories a day—for instance, reducing intake by 1,000 calories or more to lose weight faster—they should not consume less than 1,600 calories a day. Any less makes it unlikely you'll consume the essential nutrients your body needs from food. (See the "MyPyramid for Kids" section in this chapter for more on meeting a child's nutrient needs.) Plus, sticking with a minimum of 1,600 daily calories on a MyPyramid plan promotes dietary satisfaction, so you're more likely to continue eating in a healthy manner until you achieve your weight loss goals, and afterward, too.

If you want to cut fewer than 500 calories a day, that's fine, too. You will still lose weight, but you'll have to be patient because the weight will come off more slowly. It's more important to pick a safe and comfortable calorie level that's right for you than to lose weight rapidly.

Power Point _____

Adding physical activity speeds weight loss, and it can be particularly helpful for whittling down your waistline when you have no desire to make drastic cuts in calorie intake, or when you can't cut more calories for safety's sake. Physical activity has many other benefits, too. See Chapter 2 for more.

MyPyramid for Pregnancy and Nursing

Pregnant women can use a MyPyramid plan as a foundation for healthy eating. Adding calories to your baseline needs for pregnancy or nursing, and making wise choices from MyPyramid's food groups, is an excellent way to provide your baby with the nutrients it needs to grow while nourishing your body, too.

Think back to your lifestyle prior to pregnancy. Figure your daily calorie needs to maintain your weight as a woman who is not expecting or breast-feeding a child. Add 300 calories to your pre-pregnancy calorie needs for pregnancy, and add 500 calories a day to your pre-pregnancy calorie needs when nursing.

News flash: You don't actually need the extra calories for pregnancy until the second trimester begins, but go ahead and eat more if you're hungry.

Your doctor will expect you to gain between three-quarters of a pound and one pound a week from the start of the second trimester until delivery. Women who begin their pregnancies at a healthy weight and are expecting just one child should gain about 25 to 35 pounds during pregnancy; women having twins need to put on between 35 and 45 pounds.

Surveying Serving Sizes

The 12 MyPyramid eating plans make you aware of how many servings to eat each day from the food groups. To adhere to any one of the plans, you must become familiar with the recommended portions. Unfortunately, many people suffer from "portion distortion," a tendency to mistake the amount of food we'd *like* to eat for the amount we *should* eat to maintain a healthy weight.

Most of us are out of touch with the government's suggested serving sizes for foods in the MyPyramid eating plans. It's important to pay attention to servings because even slightly bigger portions can add hundreds of calories every day.

It's wise to invest in a food scale, measuring cups, and spoons. Practice weighing and measuring food to become accustomed to the amounts you need. Knowing what a portion looks like by sight can help when you dine away from home, especially because portions are out of control at most restaurants.

Discretionary Calories

With all the emphasis on building a healthy diet, you have to wonder: does MyPyramid leave any room for fun? Yes, in it's own way. Each of the 12 pyramid eating plans reserves some calories for you to spend any way you like. That part of your calorie budget is aptly called discretionary calories.

What Are Discretionary Calories?

Discretionary calories, as defined by MyPyramid, are the calories left over after accounting for the calories required to meet your nutrient needs through low-fat and no-sugar-added foods. Huh? In other words, discretionary calories are like extra cash to blow on whatever you want.

Pyramid Speak

Discretionary calories are the calories available to spend any way you like after you have met your nutrient needs.

Hold on a minute, you say. A calorie is a calorie, right? Well, yes and no. MyPyramid eating plans are set up to provide the biggest bang for your caloric buck.

The nutrition experts who designed the pyramids want you to spend the bulk of your calories getting the essential nutrients your body needs. That's why they encourage you to feast on foods such as nutrient-rich whole grain cereal for breakfast instead of high-calorie, low-nutrient cheese Danish, and why they promote salads over french fries.

A few cookies and a foot-long hot dog aren't exactly desirable choices, but they are allowable. Of course, you can also use up discretionary calories with additional servings from any of the food groups, including fruit, nuts, meat, or cheese, and by adding sauces, salad dressings, or margarine to foods.

What about alcohol? If you choose to drink alcohol, do so in moderation. Moderate drinking means up to one drink a day for women and up to two drinks for men. Twelve ounces of regular beer, five ounces of wine, or one and a half ounces of 80-proof distilled spirits count as a drink. Generally speaking, anything more than moderate drinking can be harmful to your health. And some people, or people in certain situations, shouldn't drink any alcohol at all.

Don't Go Overboard

Before you get too excited about discretionary calories, consider that it's easier than you think to spend them. In fact, going overboard on added fats, sugars, and alcohol is one of the reasons why so many Americans weigh more than they should.

Plus, the allowances for discretionary calories in all of the 12 pyramid eating plans are minimal, ranging from 100 to 300 calories. That's not much, considering a can of regular soda or 12 ounces of

beer contain about 150 calories, and two ounces of
potato chips amounts to about 300 calories. (See
Chapter 11 for more on the number of discretionary calories in each MyPyramid eating plan.)

> **Power Point**
>
> Use the Nutrition Facts panel on food
> labels to keep track of discretionary calo-
> ries. Mind your portions, however. If you
> eat more than the stated serving size, be
> sure to account for it.

Nibbling the Day Away

Struggling with your weight? Some nutrition
experts say 100 calories a day can make all the difference. You may think you're vigilant about
watching what you eat, but chances are you don't
account for extra noshing you do throughout the
day. A handful of popcorn or crackers; your child's
unfinished peanut butter and jelly sandwich; or just
two medium-size cookies and other stolen nibbles
can easily add up to 100 calories.

Head off mindless munching by chewing gum
when you feel like nibbling. Every time you want a
bite of food, you'll be forced to take out the gum to
eat. Keeping a food journal also works to deter
extra noshing as long as you write down everything
you eat and drink.

MyPyramid for Kids

By the time a child reaches two, his growth has slowed quite a bit compared to infancy. This is also the time of his life when he begins to eat what the family is eating. The beauty of the 12 MyPyramid eating plans is that you can use them to feed every member of your family over the age of two. In general, family members can eat different amounts of the same foods.

It's important to choose a plan with enough calories for your child, no matter what his age. If you are puzzled by your child's calorie needs, ask your pediatrician or a registered dietitian for advice. Never restrict your child's calories because you think he or she is too heavy. A child's rapid development translates into tremendous nutrient demands that must be met through food. Restricting food intake jeopardizes your child's development.

In Chapter 11, you may notice that the MyPyramid plans pertaining to children under age eight allow for more discretionary calories. Why? A child's nutrient needs are lower in relation to an adult's. However, that's no reason to fill up on low-nutrient foods such as candy and chips. It's best to offer a variety of nutrient-filled foods from all the food groups at meals and snacks.

The Least You Need to Know

- ◆ Calorie needs are based on age, gender, and physical activity.

- ◆ To lose weight, pick a MyPyramid plan with fewer calories, but don't go below 1,600 a day.

- ◆ You can lose weight by adding physical activity without reducing your caloric intake.

- ◆ Pay close attention to portion sizes to keep calories in line.

- ◆ Discretionary calories are yours to spend however you like.

- ◆ Children require adequate calories to grow properly, so be sure to choose a MyPyramid plan that fits their needs.

Grains

In This Chapter

- The health benefits of grains
- The best grains to eat
- New grain serving sizes
- Ways to eat healthy grains

Getting enough grains? No doubt you are. In fact, if you're like many Americans, your love of bread, pasta, and rice is making it difficult for you to shed pounds or maintain your weight. MyPyramid can help, with its fresh take on grain serving sizes and an emphasis on certain grain products that actually assist in weight control. Read on to find out what grains are most beneficial and how to make the healthiest grain choices part of your daily diet.

Grains: Divide and Conquer

Grains include food made from wheat, rice, oats, rye, cornmeal, and barley, such as bread, bagels, pasta, oatmeal and other cooked cereals, ready-to-eat breakfast cereals, tortillas, sandwich wraps, and grits.

Some grains are better than others, however. Even you know that as you're reaching for a jelly donut instead of whole wheat toast. MyPyramid separates grains into two groups—whole and refined—and emphasizes (surprise!) whole grains. Does that mean refined grains aren't worth the calories? Not necessarily.

Whole Grains

Whole grains are made from the entire grain seed known as the kernel. The kernel consists of the bran, germ, and endosperm.

Nutrition experts prefer whole grains because they retain more of their natural nutrients, including dietary fiber, B vitamins, vitamin E, and selenium.

 Pyramid Speak

> **Whole grains** contain the entire grain kernel, which includes the bran, germ, and endosperm.

MyPyramid recommends using up at least half of your Grains group allowance on whole grain foods. That amounts to a minimum of three servings daily for most adults. Young children typically need fewer whole grain servings because their grain allowance is smaller. Children should gradually increase whole grain intake as they get older, however.

Here are some examples of whole grain foods:

Whole wheat flour	Whole wheat crackers
Bulgur (cracked wheat)	Whole wheat pasta
Oatmeal	Whole grain barley
Whole grain cornmeal	Whole wheat tortillas
Brown rice	Whole grain breads
Popcorn	Millet
Whole wheat cereal flakes	Muesli
Wild rice	Quinoa

Refined Grains

Refined grains are milled. Milling removes the bran and germ from the kernel, as well as the dietary fiber, iron, and many of the B vitamins. Why strip a grain of some of its most beneficial parts? Two reasons: to give grains a finer texture and to keep them fresh longer.

Pyramid Speak

Refined grains are milled, removing the bran and germ from the kernel along with dietary fiber, iron, and many B vitamins.

Some examples of refined grain products are:

White flour	Cornbread
Degermed cornmeal	Corn Tortillas

White bread	Flour Tortillas
White rice	Crackers
Couscous	Grits
Pasta	Pretzels
Donuts*	Pastry*
Cookies*	Cake*

Ready-to-eat cereal (check the ingredients label)

Contains added sugar and fat.

There is an upside to refined grain products: most, including breakfast cereals and breads, are enriched. Enrichment is the process of adding back the B vitamins thiamin, riboflavin, and niacin, as well as the mineral iron, after processing. However, fiber levels are often lower in enriched grains than in whole grains because fiber is not added back after milling.

Enriched flour must contain folic acid, a B vitamin that helps prevent neural tube defects, a category of birth defects that occur within the first month of pregnancy. Folic acid also helps the body form red blood cells.

Power Point _____

Get the biggest bang for your nutritional buck. Check the ingredient list on refined grain products to be sure the word *enriched* is listed before the word "flour."

Great Grains

When it comes to whole grains, the whole is greater than the sum of its parts. Nutrition experts say the nutrients found in each part of the grain kernel seem to work together to provide the health benefits whole grains offer. Here are some of the many benefits whole grains, and enriched refined grains, bestow:

- Grains are a major source of carbohydrates, the body's preferred energy source.

- The B vitamins in grains——thiamin, riboflavin, niacin, and folate——play a key role in helping the body tap the energy from protein, fat, and carbohydrates. B vitamins are also essential for a healthy nervous system. Many refined grains are enriched with these B vitamins.

- As part of a healthy diet, whole grains reduce the risk of heart disease.

- Eating more whole grains than refined may foster easier weight control. The higher levels of fiber in whole grains provide feelings of fullness without adding calories.

- Foods filled with fiber, including whole grains, help reduce constipation.

- Enriched grains supply iron, used to carry oxygen in the blood. Whole and enriched refined grain products are major sources of non-heme iron for Americans, especially children.

- Whole grains are a source of selenium, a mineral that protects cells from damage, and is needed for a healthy immune system.

- The magnesium in whole grains is a mineral used in building bones and releasing energy from muscles.

Enriched refined grains are okay, but whole grains rule. How do you find whole grains on supermarket shelves? You'll see in the next section.

Hunting for Whole Grains

Many whole grain foods, including bread and brown rice, are darker than their refined counterparts. Even so, don't count on color to determine whether or not a product is a whole grain food. Food manufacturers may add darker ingredients, including molasses and colors, to give their products a darker hue. Wheat bread is a good example of how you can get hung up on a name. Most bread is made from wheat, so bread must specify that it contains whole wheat or whole grain in the ingredient list to qualify as a whole grain product.

Whole grains may or may not be rich in fiber. That's one of the reasons why you shouldn't rely solely on the grams of fiber listed in the Nutrition Facts panel. Whole grains can come from any type of grain, including wheat, oats, corn, rice, and barley, which vary in fiber content.

Some grain products, including ready-to-eat cereals, contain significant amounts of bran. Bran boosts fiber content, without providing the health benefits of whole grains. That's because bran is not a whole grain, it's just one part of the kernel.

Power Point

Foods labeled with the words multi-grain, stone-ground, 100% wheat, cracked wheat, seven-grain, and bran are usually not whole-grain products.

Go With the Whole Grain

So now you know the difference between whole and refined grains, and you're clear on why whole grains are superior. All you have to do is put whole grain advice into practice. Use these tips to make it easier to eat whole grains every day.

- Choose 100% whole grain breads, cereals, rice, pasta, and crackers.
- Add whole grains, such as barley or cracked wheat, to mixed dishes such as soups, stews, and casseroles.
- Instead of white rice, create a whole grain pilaf with a mixture of barley, wild rice, brown rice, broth, and spices. Stir in chopped dried fruit for extra flavor and nutrition.
- Substitute whole wheat flour for up to half of the white flour in your favorite quick bread recipes, including pancakes, waffles, and muffins; try working more whole wheat flour into cookie recipes, too.

- ◆ Snack on ready-to-eat, whole grain cereals such as toasted oat cereal.
- ◆ Swap snack chips for popcorn, a whole grain.

Grain Portions

If you've had any dieting experience, you may think of a grain portion as a slice of bread or a half-cup of cooked pasta. The experts who designed MyPyramid think along the same lines, with one exception.

The most recent recommendations for grains promoted by MyPyramid include a new wrinkle in portion sizes—the *ounce-equivalent*, which is the amount of food equal to a one-ounce portion of bread. No matter what calorie level you choose, you'll be advised to eat a certain number of ounce-equivalents of grains daily.

 Pyramid Speak

An **ounce-equivalent** of grains is the amount of food equal to a one-ounce slice of bread.

The following table spells out how much of some popular grain products equate to one ounce of bread.

Food	Amount equal to one-ounce equivalent
Bagels	1 mini
Biscuits	1 small (2" in diameter)
Breads	1 regular slice or 1 small slice French, or 4 snack-size slices
Bulgur	½ cup cooked
Cornbread	1 small piece (2½" × 1¼" × 1¼")
Crackers	5 whole wheat crackers or 2 rye crisp breads or 7 square or round crackers
English muffins	½ muffin
Oatmeal	½ cup cooked or 1 instant packet or 1 ounce dry (regular or quick-cooking)
Pancakes	1 pancake (4½" in diameter) or 2 small pancakes (3" in diameter)
Popcorn	3 cups popped (note: 1 microwave bag = 4 portions)
Ready-to-eat cereal	1 cup flakes or rounds or 1¼ cup puffed cereal
Rice	½ cup cooked or 1 ounce dry
Pasta	½ cup cooked or 1 ounce dry
Tortillas	1 small flour or corn tortilla (6")

Source: www.mypyramid.gov.

Servings: Size Matters

Quick. How many grain servings does your morning bagel eat up? Two, maybe three? Try about four. Sure, you have your bagel without cream cheese or butter, and that saves on calories. Unfortunately for bagel lovers, most commercial types are worth three-quarters of the daily grain allowance on the 2,000 calorie MyPyramid eating plan!

Power Point _____

Purchase two-ounce frozen bagels (equal to two ounce-equivalents from the Grains group) to prepare at home. You'll save calories and cash. Even better, choose a whole grain variety for more fiber and an array of other nutrients.

You can't plan a diet without prescribed portion sizes, like the ones the Grains group provides. And you can't stay within your calorie range without sticking to the recommended serving sizes. You've heard this before, but it bears repeating especially when it comes to foods in the Grains group: If you have no clue what a half-cup of cooked rice or bran flakes looks like, it pays to weigh and measure your food, at least for a while.

The Least You Need to Know

- ◆ Choose whole grains more often than not.

- ◆ Whole grains have more nutrients than refined grains.

- ◆ Enriched grains must contain folic acid, which fends off neural tube birth defects.

- ◆ The carbohydrates found in grains are not at the root of weight control problems; however, large portions of grains, or any food, may be.

Chapter 5

Vegetables

In This Chapter

- ◆ Meet the members of the Vegetables group and subgroups
- ◆ Discover the virtues of vegetables
- ◆ Understand vegetable serving sizes
- ◆ Uncover ways to work with vegetables

A vegetable is a vegetable, right? Yes and no. MyPyramid's Vegetables group includes your favorites as well as some you may not expect. Plus, MyPyramid goes further than its predecessor in dividing vegetables into subgroups and suggesting how much to eat from each over the course of a week. If it all sounds a bit confusing, take heart. This chapter digs into the Vegetables group and takes the mystery out of MyPyramid's vegetable recommendations.

What's in the Vegetables Group?

Under MyPyramid's direction, vegetables fall into one of five categories: Dark Green; Orange; Dried Peas and Beans (cook before eating, of course!); Starchy; and Other vegetables. The vegetables Americans tend to eat the most include foods such as potatoes, lettuce, and corn, as well as artichokes, sweet potatoes, carrots, and cauliflower. While these are all part of the Vegetables group, they belong to various subgroups within their category.

Why segregate vegetables? Although they have many common nutrients, certain vegetables provide more of particular nutrients than others. Categorizing them helps you get the nutrients you need, but only if you eat the vegetables in the recommended amounts. That may prove to be a monumental challenge for Americans, who are notorious for their inadequate vegetable intake. Perhaps if we knew more about their benefits, we'd make vegetables a priority.

Why Eat Vegetables?

Vegetables are important sources of many nutrients that promote well-being, both short- and long-term. Population studies show people who eat more fruits and vegetables as part of an overall healthy diet are less likely to develop certain chronic diseases, including heart disease, stroke, type 2 diabetes, cancer of the mouth and stomach, and colon-rectum cancer.

The Carbohydrate Connection

Vegetables provide carbohydrate for energy, and, depending on the choice, are good sources of fiber, a type of carbohydrate your body cannot digest but needs for good health nevertheless. Diets rich in foods containing fiber, such as fruits and vegetables, may reduce the risk of coronary heart disease by reducing blood cholesterol levels. And fiber is important for proper bowel function because it helps reduce constipation.

An Array of Vitamins

Vegetables and vitamins go hand in hand. The many choices from the Vegetables group supply an array of vitamins that promote good health.

Vitamin A keeps eyes and skin healthy and helps protect against infections. Vitamin E helps protect Vitamin A and essential fatty acids from damage by free radicals, troublesome forms of oxygen. Vitamin C heals cuts and wounds, bolsters teeth and gums, keeps the immune system in top shape, and boosts the absorption of iron from foods. The B vitamin folate reduces the risk of neural tube defects in developing babies and builds healthy red blood cells.

Vegetables Are All Wet

Vegetables can help satisfy your fluid requirements. Surprised? Don't be. Most vegetables are predominantly water by weight. For example, lettuce is 95 percent water; broccoli is 91 percent; and water accounts for 87 percent of a carrot's weight. Of course, vegetables and fruits are not your only sources for fluid. See Chapter 10 for more on proper hydration.

> **Fun FAQs**
>
> What do vegetables have to do with bone health? Plenty. As it turns out, strong bones require more than calcium and vitamin D. The vitamin K present in dark green leafy vegetables, such as kale and broccoli, is central to bone strength. Vegetables are also a bounty of potassium and magnesium, minerals that help bones retain the calcium they need to resist fracture.

Vegetable Variety

MyPyramid emphasizes eating an array of vegetables every day. It also recommends weekly minimums for different types of vegetables.

Each of the 12 MyPyramid plans includes a prescribed number of total vegetable servings per day and advice on how many servings to eat from each vegetable subgroup on a weekly basis. (See the "Eat

Your Veggies!" section later in this chapter for an example of how it works on a 2,000 calorie-a-day plan.)

The following sections list groups of vegetables and their subgroupings.

Dark Green Vegetables

Dark green vegetables include:

- Broccoli
- Bok choy
- Collard greens
- Dark green leafy lettuce
- Kale
- Watercress
- Mesclun
- Mustard greens
- Romaine lettuce
- Spinach
- Turnip greens

Orange Vegetables

Orange vegetables include:

- Acorn squash
- Butternut squash
- Carrots
- Hubbard squash
- Pumpkin
- Sweet potatoes

Dry Beans and Peas

Cooked, dry beans and peas include:

- Black beans
- Black-eyed peas
- Garbanzo beans (chickpeas)
- Navy beans
- Pinto beans
- Soybeans

- Kidney beans
- Lentils
- Lima beans (mature)

- Split peas
- White beans
- Tofu (bean curd made from soybeans)

Starchy Vegetables

Starchy vegetables include:

- Corn
- Green peas

- Lima beans
- Potatoes

Other Vegetables

Other vegetables include:

- Artichokes
- Asparagus
- Bean sprouts
- Beets
- Brussels sprouts
- Cabbage
- Cauliflower
- Celery
- Cucumbers
- Eggplant
- Green beans
- Green and red sweet peppers

- Iceberg (head) lettuce
- Mushrooms
- Okra
- Onions
- Parsnips
- Tomatoes
- Tomato juice*
- Vegetable juice*
- Turnips
- Wax beans
- Zucchini

May be high in sodium.

Sizing Up Vegetables

Any vegetable or 100% vegetable juice is a member of the Vegetables group. Vegetables may be raw or cooked; fresh, frozen, canned, or dried/dehydrated; and may be whole, cut-up, or mashed.

When cooking vegetables, lightly steam or microwave them to preserve nutrient content; this also allows for certain nutrients, including fiber, and disease-fighting carotenoids found in dark green and orange vegetables, to be more available to your body for absorption. Grilling and roasting are also worthy cooking methods for vegetables, as long as you don't overcook them.

If your idea of a serving of vegetables is the lettuce and the lone tomato slice on a fast-food burger, you're in for a shock.

Generally speaking, 1 cup of raw or cooked vegetables or vegetable juice, or 2 cups of raw leafy greens, is considered a vegetable serving.

The following table lists specific amounts that count as 1 cup of vegetables.

Food	Amount that counts as 1 cup of vegetables
Dark Green Vegetables	
Broccoli	1 cup chopped or florets 3 spears 5" long, raw or cooked
Greens: collard, mustard, turnip, kale, cooked greens	1 cup cooked
Raw leafy greens: spinach, romaine, watercress, dark green leafy lettuce, endive, escarole	2 cups raw
Orange Vegetables	
Carrots	1 cup, strips, slices, or chopped, raw or cooked 2 medium whole
	1 cup baby carrots (about 12)
Pumpkin	1 cup mashed, cooked
Sweet potato	1 large baked (2¼" or more in diameter) 1 cup sliced or mashed, cooked
Winter squash	1 cup cubed, cooked (acorn, butternut, hubbard)
Dry Beans and Peas	
Dry beans and peas	1 cup whole or mashed, cooked (includes black, garbanzo, kidney, pinto, or soy bean, black-eyed peas or split peas, lentils)
Tofu	1 cup (½" cubes), about 8 ounces

Food	Amount that counts as 1 cup of vegetables
Starchy Vegetables	
Corn, yellow or white	1 cup 1 large ear (8" to 9" long)
Green peas	1 cup
Potatoes	1 cup diced, mashed 1 medium boiled or baked (2½" to 3" in diameter) French fried: 20 medium to long strips (2½" to 4" long)
Other Vegetables	
Bean sprouts	1 cup cooked
Cabbage, green	1 cup chopped or shredded, raw or cooked
Cauliflower	1 cup pieces of florets, raw or cooked
Celery	1 cup diced or sliced, raw or cooked or 2 large stalks (11" to 12" long)
Cucumbers	1 cup sliced, chopped, or raw
Green or wax beans	1 cup cooked
Lettuce, iceberg	2 cups raw, shredded or chopped or a head
Mushrooms	1 cup raw or cooked
Onions	1 cup chopped, raw or cooked
Tomatoes	1 large whole raw, 3" 1 cup chopped or sliced, raw, canned or cooked
Tomato or mixed vegetable juice	1 cup
Summer squash or zucchini	1 cup cooked, sliced or diced

Source: www.mypyramid.gov.

Sprouts may be on MyPyramid's vegetable list, but they shouldn't be on your plate. In the last 10 years, hundreds of people in the U.S. have become ill from eating raw and cooked sprouts, including alfalfa, clover, and mung bean, but not Brussels sprouts. In spite of a concerted effort by government and industry to ensure sprout safety, contamination has not decreased, prompting the Food and Drug Administration to warn everyone off sprouts of any sort.

Eat Your Veggies!

Eat your veggies, they're good for you! You heard that a million times as a child, and you're hearing it now. Of course, nutrition experts know more now than your mother did about why vegetables promote good health, but it's all the same in the end.

MyPyramid's Vegetables group is probably the hardest of all the food groups to decipher. Although it may be difficult at first, the more you use the plan, the easier it becomes to work in the required vegetables.

Here's how the vegetable recommendations break down on the 2,000 calorie pyramid plan:

Total daily vegetable servings needed: 2½ cups

Over the course of a week, eat:

- 3 cups dark green vegetables
- 2 cups orange vegetables
- 3 cups dried beans and peas
- 3 cups starchy vegetables
- 6½ cups other vegetables

Wow, that seems like a lot of produce, doesn't it? It can be overwhelming to see the requirements, but remember, this is over the course of seven days. Including vegetables at lunch and dinner is one way of getting the recommended amounts.

Don't worry and don't give up if you don't satisfy all the requirements in the first week of using the plan. Remember MyPyramid's slogan, *Steps to a Healthier You*, encourages small changes toward a healthier lifestyle.

Ways to Work Vegetables Into Your Diet

Including vegetables can mean more than steaming broccoli for dinner or having a limp iceberg salad with a few slices of cucumber for lunch. There are dozens of ways to incorporate vegetables into meals and snacks. Here are some suggestions that are sure to appeal to veggie-resistant adults and children alike:

- Make vegetables part of soups, casseroles, meatloaf, and pasta dishes. For example, add chopped frozen kale to homemade or low-sodium canned soup. You won't even notice it's there.

- Serve raw, sliced vegetables with peanut butter, hummus, or low-fat salad dressing for dipping.

- Make vegetables available and tasty. Half the battle is having them in the house and ready to eat.

- Purchase fresh vegetables in season. They typically taste better and are less costly.

- Stock up on frozen vegetables in bags so you can take what you need without waste. Plain frozen vegetables are preferable to canned because they are far lower in sodium.

- For the sake of convenience, purchase pre-washed salad greens and other chopped vegetables to make preparation a snap.

- Add baby carrots or grape tomatoes to your lunch or take them with you to work or daytime activities as a readily available snack.

- Make vegetables the star attraction in a tofu-vegetable stir-fry dish. Marinate firm tofu in low-sodium salad dressing or low-sodium soy sauce for extra flavor.

- Eat salad for a meal, and don't forget a source of protein, which could be beans, tofu, poultry, or seafood. Go easy on the full-fat salad dressing.

- Make it a habit to include a green salad and at least one other vegetable for dinner every night.

- Choose bean-based soups and stews, such as lentil and vegetarian chili, instead of chicken noodle.

- Keep canned beans on hand to add to salads, soups, and pasta dishes or to eat as a snack.

- Snack on salsa, hummus, or black bean dip and baked snack chips made from toasted whole wheat pita bread.

- Grow a garden and enlist the help of your child.

- Include chopped vegetables in prepared pasta sauce or your favorite lasagna dish.

- Use pureéd, cooked vegetables such as potatoes to thicken stews, soups, and gravies.
These add flavor, nutrients, and texture.

- Allow older children to help shop for, clean,
peel, or cut up vegetables.

- When shopping, encourage children to pick
a new vegetable to try at home.

- Keep feeding vegetables to kids. Children
may need to be exposed to a food upwards
of 10 times before they accept it.

- Trade off textures to keep vegetables interesting. Substitute roasted carrots for
steamed, and raw broccoli for cooked.

As you use a MyPyramid plan, you'll come up with
your own ways of making vegetables a part of your
daily diet.

So, You're Not Into Veggies

Do you gag at the thought of broccoli or want to
run when served anything but potatoes and corn?
For you, variety is not the spice of life. Of course,
it would be wonderful if you chose lentil soup
instead of chicken noodle; opted for spinach over
iceberg lettuce; and munched on raw carrots and
celery. Alas, you probably won't.

But you do like some vegetables, so let's work with
that. It's better to eat more of the vegetables you
favor to reach your daily quota than giving up on
getting there. That's because any vegetable is better
than none, even though variety is one of the major
tenets of MyPyramid eating plans.

Power Point _____

> Try adding some fat, such as olive oil or cheese sauce, to vegetables to make them more attractive and better for you. A recent study found your body won't absorb some of the disease-fighting nutrients that vegetables have to offer without some fat at the same meal. Go easy, however. Gobs of butter or margarine are not advised.

Can you substitute fruit for vegetables? Yes, some of the time.

But you should try to learn to like a wider variety of vegetables. Don't go on the memory of mom's limp green beans and canned carrots. The vegetables you rejected as a teenager may hold great appeal for you now, especially when prepared in a flavorful way.

The Least You Need to Know

- ◆ Vegetables provide an array of health benefits.
- ◆ MyPyramid's Vegetables group includes dry beans and peas.
- ◆ Vegetables fall into one of five subcategories within the Vegetables group in the MyPyramid eating plans.
- ◆ You should eat a certain amount of vegetables from each subgroup over a week's time.
- ◆ Vegetables can contribute significant fluid to your diet.

Chapter 6

Fruits

In This Chapter

- Why fruit is good for you
- How much fruit to eat every day
- Why you and your kids should limit juices
- How to make fruit part of your day

Whew! You made it through the chapter on vegetables. With any luck, you're not too exhausted to continue on. Luckily, MyPyramid's fruit recommendations are much easier to swallow than the ones for vegetables.

This chapter explains the healthy rewards of fruit as part of a balanced diet; how much fruit is enough; and suggests new ways to eat your favorite fruits.

Why Eat Fruit?

Besides the fact that fruit tastes great, there are myriad health reasons for including fruit in your daily diet. Like vegetables, fruit provides an array of nutrients. Fruits supply carbohydrates, vitamins, minerals, fiber, potassium, and water. See Chapter 5 for more on these nutrients.

Almost all fruit is naturally low in fat, sodium, and calories. Fruit does not contain cholesterol and has no protein to speak of. A diet rich in fruits and vegetables as part of an overall healthy diet may reduce your risk for:

- Stroke and other cardiovascular diseases, such as heart disease
- Type 2 diabetes
- Mouth, stomach, and colon-rectum cancer
- Bone loss
- Kidney stones

Eating foods, such as fruit, that are low in calories instead of other higher-calorie sweet treats, including cake, candy, and cookies, may be useful in helping keep calories under control. Although fruit is not as low in calories as many vegetables, it is a wiser choice. Fruit contains fiber and water, two food components that contribute to eating satisfaction without adding calories. (Plus, fiber and water ward off constipation, too.)

Eating more fresh fruit is linked to a lower weight in children. Research shows children who munch on fruit have a lower Body Mass Index. Eating fruit also crowds out other higher calorie, low-nutrient foods in a child's diet.

Fruits and Phytonutrients

Ellagic acid. Carotenoids. Isoflavones. Nutrition experts fling these words around when talking about fruits and vegetables. What are they talking about?

They are *phytonutrients*, also known as phytochemicals—which are any chemical found in a plant—including fruits, vegetables, grains, and legumes. Neither vitamins nor minerals, the thousands of phytonutrients in plant foods play a role in promoting health.

Pyramid Speak _____

Phytonutrients, whose root is phyto, comes from the Greek word *phyton* (plant). Phytonutrients mean plant nutrients.

Scientists suspect phytonutrients help fight off chronic conditions, including cataracts, cancer, and heart disease. Certain phytonutrients are antioxidants that ward off cell damage that could be the beginnings of disease. Still others stimulate anticancer enzymes in the body, while some phytonutrients whisk potential cancer-starting agents out of your body.

Fruit Medley

Sure, you get the fruit you need every day. But are you satisfying MyPyramid's variety recommendation? Here's how to take fruit consumption to the next level.

Mix It Up

You top your morning cereal with sliced banana and you munch on an apple for a snack at some point during the day. You should be congratulated for satisfying the fruit quota on a 2,000 calorie MyPyramid eating plan. You're ahead of most people and you're ready for more variety.

When you expand your fruit choices, you may be rewarded with even greater health benefits. Swapping the banana for a half-cup of blueberries gets you far more antioxidants, a type of substance in plant foods that thwarts cell damage (see the previous section on Fruits and Phytonutrients for more). And munching on a handful of dried cranberries instead of an apple every day may help ward off urinary tract infections in women. Cranberries contain a substance that thwarts bacterial growth in the urinary tract.

Are apples and bananas bad? On the contrary. Bananas and apples offer their own benefits. Getting stuck in a nutrition rut may work against you, however.

The Juicy Details

What about drinking juice as an option to whole fruit? Juice is loaded with vitamins, minerals, and phytonutrients. However, 100% juice drinks lack the fiber of whole fruits. Fiber is filling. That's why it's so much easier to down eight ounces of orange juice—with about 100 calories and a half-gram of fiber—than it is to eat an orange for about 70 calories and nearly four grams of fiber.

Kids gravitate toward sweet beverages, and parents may think of juice as the answer to regular soda and other sugary soft drinks. It's not, exactly. The American Academy of Pediatrics recommends limiting a child's juice intake to just six ounces (three-quarters cup) a day until he's six years old. The high natural sugar content of juice can cause diarrhea in otherwise healthy children. Plus, because juice is so easy to drink without filling up and it's a concentrated calorie source, juice can easily interfere with weight control in kids and adults.

Pitfalls

Avoid juice concoctions with the terms cocktail, drink, beverage, and any word ending in -ade (such as lemonade) on the front of the label. They contain less than 100% juice and are not worthy. Drink only pasteurized juice for safety's sake. Check the label to be sure.

Fruit Portions

Any fruit from apples to watermelon to 100% fruit juice counts as part of MyPyramid's Fruits group. Fruits may be fresh, canned, frozen, or dried, and may be whole, cut-up, or pureéd. The following table provides fruit serving guidelines.

Fruit	Amount that counts as 1 cup of fruit
Apple	½ large (3¼" diameter) 1 small (2½" diameter) or 1 cup sliced or chopped, raw or cooked
Applesauce	1 cup
Banana	1 large (8"–9") or 1 cup sliced
Berries (blueberries, raspberries, blackberries, etc.)	1 cup
Cantaloupe	1 cup diced or melon balls
Grapes	1 cup whole or cut-up or 32 seedless grapes
Grapefruit	1 medium (4" in diameter) or 1 cup sections
Mixed fruit (fruit cocktail)	1 cup
Orange	1 large (about 3" in diameter) or 1 cup sections
Orange, mandarin	1 cup canned, drained
Peach	1 large (2¾" in diameter) or 1 cup sliced or diced, raw, cooked or canned, drained or 2 halves, canned

Fruit	Amount that counts as 1 cup of fruit
Pear	1 medium pear (2½ per pound) or 1 cup sliced or diced, raw, cooked, or canned, drained
Pineapple	1 cup chunks, sliced or crushed, raw, cooked or canned, drained
Plum	3 medium or 2 large plums or 1 cup sliced raw or cooked
Strawberries	About 8 large berries or 1 cup whole, halved, or sliced, fresh or frozen
Watermelon	1 small wedge (1" thick) or 1 cup diced or balls
Dried fruit (apricots, blueberries, cherries, cranberries, prunes, and so on)	¼ cup of dried fruit
100% fruit juice	1 cup

Source: www.mypyramid.gov.

Focus on Fruit

Fitting in fruit is far less complicated than you may think. All it takes is a bit of planning to keep fruit front and center in your diet. Of course, shopping for fruit on a regular basis is a must, but there are so many other ways to keep fruit on hand that you won't have any excuses to exclude fruit, even if your life is hectic and you're not always home for meals.

This list provides suggestions for incorporating fruit; fighting fruit boredom; and ways to keep you, and your children, interested in eating a variety of fruits every day.

- Keep fruit on hand at home and at work. You can't eat fruit if it's not available.

- Place fruit, such as bananas, in a bowl in plain sight so that children and adults will be more apt to grab fruit instead of sugary or fatty snacks.

- Purchase seasonal fruits for better taste and higher quality. Try clementines from Spain during the winter as a change from oranges and tangerines.

- Stock up on dried fruits, including cranberries, raisins, and apricots; frozen varieties, such as berries and melon; and canned fruit, including mandarin oranges, peaches, pears, and pineapple canned in water or juice.

- Pick pre-cut packages of fruit (such as melon or pineapple chunks) for added convenience. To get more for your money, buy the whole fruit and cut it up yourself.

- Choose whole fruit, including apples and oranges, instead of their juice.

- Select fruits with higher potassium more often, such as bananas, prunes and prune juice, dried peaches and apricots, cantaloupe, honeydew melon, and orange juice.

- Top breakfast cereal with berries, bananas, or dried fruit.

- Offer children frozen fruit, including melon chunks and bananas. Frozen fruit adds an element of fun.

- Add berries to pancakes.

- Opt for 100% orange or grapefruit juice over juice drinks.

- Pack fruit with your lunch and to have as snacks. When you're on the go, tote dried fruit in your car or briefcase.

- Add chopped green or red seedless grapes to chicken salad.

- For something different, add crushed pineapple to coleslaw, or toss salad greens with mandarin oranges, dried cranberries, cherries, or blueberries, or chopped grapes.

- Prepare a fruit crisp or baked apples for dessert or snack. Dried figs and dates are also sweet, ready-to-eat treats.

- Stir dried fruit into cooked oatmeal or other hot cereal.

- Prepare a peanut butter and banana sandwich on whole wheat bread.

- Spread almond butter on sliced apples or pears.

- Pureé canned fruits, such as apricots or berries, and use it to top or combine with low-fat or fat-free yogurt.

- Opt for frozen 100% juice bars instead of high-fat frozen treats.

- Provide kids with low-fat yogurt for dipping sliced fruit.

- Offer children applesauce or other fruit pureé for dipping French toast slices or pancakes.

- Make a fruit salad to have on hand. Toss with lemon or orange juice to keep fruit from turning brown.

- Allow children to be involved in choosing and preparing fruit. Let them explore the fruit section of the supermarket and allow them to choose a new fruit to try at home.

- Offer raisins or other dried fruits instead of candy. Make your own trail mix with dried fruit, ready-to-eat cereal, and chopped nuts. (Children under age 4 should not eat dried fruit or nuts because they are choking risks.)

- Assemble fruit kabobs using pineapple chunks, bananas, grapes, and berries.

- Always include fruit when dining at fast food chains or restaurants. If no cut fruit is available, order 100% fruit juice.

Power Point

Homemade banana smoothies combine a serving each of fruit and dairy for dessert or snack. Combine a ripe banana, eight ounces of low fat milk or yogurt, and 2 ice cubes in a blender or food processor. Whip until frothy. Serve immediately.

The Least You Need to Know

- Fruit supplies an array of nutrients that promote good health.

- Fruit is a healthy alternative to high-fat, sweet treats.

- Kids and adults should limit juice consumption.

- Phytonutrients present in fruits and vegetables help fight off chronic conditions.

Chapter 7

Milk

In This Chapter

- Discover why milk matters
- Find out how much dairy you need daily
- Account for discretionary calories
- Discover new ways to eat dairy foods
- Learn about dairy alternatives

Perhaps you're a milk lover and you won't go a day without at least a few tall cold glasses of the stuff. Maybe you can't stand milk or any food made from it. Maybe you love it, but your body is lactose intolerant or allergic. Or it could be that you're on the fence: you tolerate dairy foods because you know they are good for you, but you don't make them a high priority.

Whatever the case, it's hard to ignore the array of nutrients MyPyramid's milk products provide when you see them explained in this chapter. Milk lovers will rejoice at the many ways to work in the suggested amounts of milk, cheese, and yogurt that follow. And those who avoid milk for any reason will find healthy alternatives in the pages ahead.

More Than Milk

Calcium is the kingpin nutrient when it comes to the Milk group. While the suggested dairy foods listed in MyPyramid's Milk category contain about the same amount of calcium as milk, serving sizes vary.

Following are some commonly consumed foods featured in the Milk group:

Milk:

- Fat-free (skim)
- Reduced-fat (2%)
- Flavored milks
- Lactose-free milk
- Low-fat (1%)
- Whole milk
- Lactose-reduced milk

Yogurt:

- Fat-free
- Reduced-fat
- Low-fat
- Whole milk

Milk-based desserts:

- Puddings made with milk
- Frozen yogurt
- Ice cream
- Ice milk

Cheese:

Hard natural cheeses:

- Cheddar
- Swiss
- Mozzarella, part-skim
- Parmesan

Soft cheeses:

+ Ricotta   + Cottage cheese

Processed cheeses:

+ American

Milk Group Portions

MyPyramid's Milk group has the easiest recommendations to remember of all the food groups. Children from ages two to eight require two cups of milk a day or the equivalent in dairy foods; after nine, the quota is three cups a day.

Power Point _____

Pregnant women do not require more than three servings of milk on a MyPyramid eating plan. That's because the body boosts its calcium absorption from foods during pregnancy to make up for the calcium the baby takes from mom's bones to develop.

Each of the following milk product servings counts as one cup.

Food	Amount equal to one cup milk
Milk	1 cup, any fat level, or ½ cup evaporated or 1 half-pint container
Yogurt	1 regular container (8 fluid ounces) or 1 cup
Cheese	1½ ounces hard cheese, such as American, cheddar, mozzarella, Swiss, and Parmesan ⅓ cup shredded cheese, 2 ounces processed cheese, ½ cup ricotta cheese, or 2 cups cottage cheese
Milk-based desserts	1 cup pudding made with milk 1 cup frozen yogurt 1½ cups ice cream

Source: www.MyPyramid.gov.

Dairy and Discretionary Calories

Some of the selections in the previous table may come as a surprise. No, your eyes have not deceived you: cheese and ice cream are allowed on any of MyPyramid's eating plans. That's not so shocking, considering that MyPyramid is all about balance.

If you're salivating just thinking about all the full-fat cheddar cheese and frozen desserts you'll eat to make your daily dairy quota, you need a reality check. For the most part, MyPyramid encourages

food choices with the least fat and added sugars
from each of the food groups to help you stay
within your given calorie budget and to foster good
health. It's no different for dairy foods.

Being Dense Is Good

When it comes to the dairy products, fat-free and
low-fat milk, fat-free and low-fat yogurt, and
reduced-fat cheeses are the most beneficial because
they are the most nutrient-dense of all the dairy
foods. *Nutrient-dense foods* provide substantial
amounts of vitamins and minerals for relatively few
calories.

Pyramid Speak

Nutrient-dense foods are those that provide substantial amounts of vitamins and
minerals and relatively few calories.

For example, eight ounces of fat-free milk supplies
about 300 milligrams of calcium for about 110
calories. To get the same calcium from vanilla ice
cream, you'd need to eat one and a half cups. That
doesn't sound so bad, until you consider the calories in that much vanilla ice cream: 425. Choosing
ice cream over fat-free milk would eat up nearly
one-quarter of most adults' daily calorie allowances.

Accounting for Extra Calories

That doesn't mean vanilla ice cream, or any other food from the Milk group, is off limits. However, when you choose milk or yogurt that is not plain and fat-free, or cheese that is not reduced-fat, you must count the extra calories the product provides as part of your discretionary calorie allowance.

The concept of discretionary calories is perhaps one of the most confusing tenets of MyPyramid, and one of the most important ones. Discretionary calories are discussed in Chapter 2.

Here's how a few grams of fat here and there in dairy foods makes a big difference in calorie consumption. With just 85 calories and 0 fat grams, fat-free milk contains no discretionary calories. Whole milk is a different story. It supplies 145 calories per cup; 65 of them are considered discretionary. The more than seven grams of fat in the whole milk is responsible for the 65-calorie difference between fat-free and whole milk. Switching from three servings of whole milk to fat-free milk shaves nearly 200 calories a day.

Choosing lower fat dairy foods goes beyond calorie-counting, however. Full-fat dairy foods, including milk, cheese, and ice cream, contain more saturated fat and cholesterol. Too much saturated fat and cholesterol from foods may increase your risk of heart disease by raising blood cholesterol levels. (Learn more about fat and cholesterol in Chapter 9.)

It may be easiest to figure discretionary calories in dairy foods by using the chart that follows as a reference. Refer to the Nutrient Facts panel on food labels to help you compute the extra calories you consume from dairy foods with more fat and added sugar.

Food	Calories
Fat-free milk, 8 ounces	85
Plain fat-free yogurt, 1 cup	137
Reduced-fat cheddar cheese, 1½ ounces	74

What if you can't stomach reduced-fat cheese and your child insists upon strawberry milk or none at all? There is a case to be made for some sugar and fat in your diet, especially when they help you to work in nutrient-dense dairy foods. Remember, discretionary calories are yours to spend any way you like.

Fun FAQs

Does your favorite coffee drink double as a serving from the Milk group? Yes, as long as you prefer lattes and cappuccinos to sugar- and fat-laden coffee smoothies. Twelve ounces of café latte or cappuccino supply between 300 and 400 milligrams of calcium, about the amount in a serving of milk. Keep calories low with fat-free milk. And opt for decaf for the healthiest drink.

Milk Matters

Think milk, and calcium comes to mind. That's reasonable. Dairy foods supply the lion's share of calcium in the American diet. Focusing solely on calcium doesn't do justice to milk's powerful overall nutrient package, however. Milk supplies a number of essential nutrients, including several vitamins and minerals.

The 2005 Dietary Guidelines for Americans identify seven nutrients that American adults and children are lacking, including calcium, potassium, magnesium, and vitamin A. Dairy foods can help make up for those nutrient shortfalls, and more. The following list highlights the many nutrients milk has to offer, and what role they play in the body:

- Protein provides the raw materials for building, repairing, and maintaining cells, tissues, and organs.

- Carbohydrates supply energy.

- Calcium builds bones and teeth and keeps them strong throughout your lifetime.

- Potassium helps maintain healthy blood pressure and normal muscle function.

- Vitamin D regulates levels of calcium and phosphorous, helping to build and maintain bones.

- Vitamin A keeps skin healthy, regulates the immune system, and helps your eyes see normally in the dark.

- Riboflavin assists in energy production for all the cells in your body.

- Niacin facilitates the normal function of enzymes in the body.

- Vitamin B12 works closely with folate to make red blood cells; plays a role in cell growth and division; and wards off nerve cell damage.

- Phosphorus collaborates with calcium to keep bones strong.

How Milk Benefits Your Health

Calcium garners the most attention when it comes to milk's nutrient package, and rightfully so. No single nutrient is the magic bullet, however. The nutrients in milk have a synergistic effect when it comes to promoting wellness. In the case of milk, and other dairy foods, the whole is greater than the sum of its parts.

Milk Bolsters Bones

Drinking milk and eating yogurt and cheese can help reduce the risk of osteoporosis, a bone-crippling disease that affects 28 million Americans, most of them women. Osteoporosis is a disease that makes bones brittle and puts you at risk for fracture.

Osteoporosis is often characterized as a pediatric disease with geriatric consequences. That's because it takes a lifetime of unhealthy habits to develop osteoporosis, a silent condition that makes itself known after midlife. Getting enough milk and milk products during childhood and adolescence, when the majority of bone mass is built, is one way to help head off osteoporosis later in life.

Milk Heads off High Blood Pressure

Low-fat dairy products assist in keeping blood pressure levels in check. The DASH (Dietary Approaches to Stop Hypertension) diet—a low-fat, calcium-rich eating plan that emphasizes low-fat dairy foods, fruits, vegetables, grains, and lean meat—has been shown in scientific studies to substantially and quickly reduce blood pressure in people with high blood pressure. The DASH diet also reduces other heart disease risk factors, including total cholesterol levels, and lowers the risk of stroke and osteoporosis.

Milk and Girth Control

A growing body of scientific evidence shows that when you include three servings of milk, yogurt, or cheese a day as part of a reduced-calorie diet, you may be able to lose more total weight and body fat than if you forego dairy foods. Studies suggest that the mix of nutrients found in milk, such as calcium and protein, may crank up the body's ability to burn fat——particularly around your midsection.

When it comes to children and teens, research has linked diets rich in calcium from milk with less abdominal fat. A study of nearly 100 children ages three through 13 who were followed for 12 years suggests that low milk consumption during childhood may contribute to gaining excess body fat as kids age.

Vitamin D: Calcium's Silent Partner

Calcium owes much of its success to vitamin D. Vitamin D promotes calcium absorption from foods and maintains proper levels of blood calcium by allowing the movement of calcium in and out of bones.

In that capacity, it heads off osteoporosis as well as osteomalacia, a bone-wasting condition characterized by chronic bone pain, muscle aches, and muscle weakness that may be incorrectly diagnosed as fibromyalgia. In children, vitamin D thwarts rickets, a bone-deforming disease.

Pitfalls

Cheese is typically made from milk that does not contain vitamin D, however. Only certain brands of yogurt contain vitamin D, so check the label to make fortified yogurt one of your Milk group choices.

Vitamin D is known as the sunshine vitamin because strong summer sunlight initiates the production of vitamin D in your skin. Sunshine is, by design, the primary vitamin D "source." In nature's grand scheme, we would produce all the vitamin D we needed and store it in fat cells for future use. However, many Americans don't make enough vitamin D for two reasons: inadequate sunshine during the winter months and sunscreen use. Slathering on sunscreen with an SPF of 8 or higher blocks beneficial rays and prevents your body from producing vitamin D.

Which brings us to why it's so important to get the vitamin D you need from foods, such as milk. Nearly all the milk sold in the United States is fortified with vitamin D. Vitamin D is also added to other foods including breads, cereals, and orange juice. Some brands of orange juice supply as much vitamin D as milk. Check the Nutrient Facts panel to see whether a food contains 25% of the Daily Value for vitamin D. That's as much vitamin D as eight ounces of milk, so it's worthy.

Dairy Dilemma

You love dairy, but it doesn't love you back. Must you forgo the pleasures of milk, yogurt, and cheese? That depends on your situation. When you can't stomach dairy, it's usually for one of two reasons. Read on for more information.

Milk Allergy

When you're allergic to milk, all dairy foods provoke a reaction that involves your immune system.

A food allergy is an overreaction of the immune system to an *allergen*, a protein in foods that the allergic person's body interprets as harmful.

Pyramid Speak

Allergens are proteins found in foods not broken down during cooking or digestion that trigger the body's immune response.

People with a milk allergy should stay away from dairy foods or look for an alternative.

The good news about milk allergy in children is that it may disappear, typically by age four. As a child's digestive tract matures, he'll absorb fewer allergens into his blood stream and his immune system will become stronger, preventing allergens from wreaking havoc on his body. Talk with your pediatrician or allergist about re-introducing your child to milk as he gets older.

Lactose Intolerance

Does your stomach churn after you drink milk, eat yogurt, or munch on a grilled cheese? You may have *lactose intolerance*.

Pyramid Speak

Lactose intolerance is a condition where your body does not make enough lactase, the enzyme necessary to break down lactose, the carbohydrate found in dairy foods.

In lactose intolerance, your body can't produce adequate amounts of lactase. Lactase is the digestive enzyme responsible for breaking down lactose, the carbohydrate found naturally in milk, yogurt, cheese, and in other dairy foods. The resulting gas, bloating, and diarrhea that may occur when lactose goes undigested causes discomfort, although symptoms pass within hours and are not considered serious.

Not everyone who is lactose intolerant reacts the same way to dairy foods. That's because lactose intolerance is not an all-or-nothing condition. Some people may be able to tolerate certain dairy foods and not others. Here are some strategies for including dairy foods that may help.

- Consume small amounts of milk products throughout the day along with other foods to mitigate the effects of lactose. For example, drink two ounces of milk during meals instead of the typical eight.

- Choose yogurt with active cultures. Active cultures break down some of the lactose for you.

- Opt for aged cheeses, such as cheddar and mozzarella, over processed cheeses. Aged cheeses contain the least lactose.

Lactose-free and lower-lactose dairy products are widely available and are excellent options for people with lactose intolerance. Lactose-free and lower-lactose dairy foods are made from milk and provide the same nutritional value. Enzyme preparations that break down lactose can be added to milk to lower the lactose content.

Make It Milk, Cheese, or Yogurt

Dairy foods are incredibly versatile. Don't like to drink milk straight up? Use milk on cereal or make fruit smoothies with milk or yogurt. You can even sneak milk into soups. Following are just a few ways to satisfy your milk quota:

- Include milk as a beverage at meals, including when you're dining out. Choose fat-free or low-fat milk.
- Prepare oatmeal and other cooked cereals with fat-free or low-fat milk.
- Make your own low fat pizza: top toasted whole grain pita bread with tomato sauce or fresh sliced tomato and reduced-fat mozzarella cheese. Broil until cheese is just melted.
- Prepare mashed potatoes, macaroni and cheese, and condensed cream soup, such as cream of tomato, with condensed milk instead of regular.

- Snack on fat-free or low-fat yogurt as a snack.

- Make your own fruit yogurt by combining fat-free or low-fat plain yogurt with a serving of fruit.

- Use fat-free or low-fat yogurt for dips instead of full-fat sour cream.

- Prepare pudding with fat-free or low-fat milk.

- Top a baked potato with fat-free or low-fat yogurt.

- Top chopped fruit with yogurt for a filling dessert or snack.

- Top casseroles, soups, stews, or vegetables with shredded low-fat cheese.

- Mix fat-free or low-fat cottage cheese with chopped fruit or berries.

- Add a slice of reduced-fat cheese to a sandwich.

- Sprinkle feta cheese on salads or use in omelets.

- Feast on fruit and cheese for dessert.

- Top pancakes with a mixture of yogurt and fruit.

- Top a toasted whole wheat bagel or 2 slices whole wheat toast with ½ cup cottage or ricotta cheese. Top with a mixture of cinnamon and sugar or a touch of jelly or jam.

- Stir ricotta cheese or cottage cheese into warm or cold pasta dishes, including pasta with marinara sauce or macaroni salad. Add ¼ cup cheese per serving.

- Mix 2 cups cottage cheese with 1 cup thick and chunky salsa and serve with chips made from toasted whole wheat pita bread.

- Scoop out the inside of a baked potato and mix with 1 cup cottage cheese. Return to potato skin shell and serve.

For more easy and delicious ways to work dairy foods into your diet, visit www.3ADay.org.

You Don't Do Dairy

If you avoid milk because of milk allergy, or because you choose not to consume dairy for other reasons, you must make an effort to replace the nutrients missing when you cut out an entire food group. Plant foods rich in calcium, and calcium-added foods are a great place to start.

That said, the body's ability to absorb calcium from plant products is not as good as for dairy foods. Some plant foods have calcium that is well absorbed, but the large quantity of plant foods that would be needed to provide as much calcium as a glass of milk may be unachievable for many people. For instance, you'd need to eat 7 cups of chopped broccoli to get the calcium in one cup of milk.

Pitfalls

Plant foods are a poor source of vitamin D. If you don't drink milk, make sure you take a multivitamin with 100% of the Daily Value for vitamin D every day.

The following table provides information about the calcium content in certain nondairy foods.

Food, Standard Amount	Calcium (milligrams)
Fortified ready-to-eat cereals, 1 oz	236–1043
Soy beverage, calcium fortified, 1 cup	368
Sardines, Atlantic, in oil, drained, 3 oz	325
Tofu, firm, prepared with nigarib, ½ cup	253
Pink salmon, canned, with bone, 3 oz	181
Collards, cooked from frozen, ½ cup	178
Molasses, blackstrap, 1 TB	172
Spinach, cooked from frozen, ½ cup	146
Soybeans, green, cooked, ½ cup	130
Turnip greens, cooked from frozen, ½ cup	124
Ocean perch, Atlantic, cooked, 3 oz	116
Oatmeal, plain and flavored, instant, fortified, 1 packet prepared	99–110
Cowpeas, cooked, ½ cup	106

Source: 2005 Dietary Guidelines for Americans.

Soy beverages and tofu processed with calcium are among the best dairy alternatives because they provide protein that goes missing when you do not include the recommended amounts of dairy on a MyPyramid eating plan. Plus, soy beverages are often fortified with calcium, vitamin D, and many of the other nutrients milk provides. Check the food label to be sure.

The Least You Need to Know

- Milk products provide an array of nutrients that promote good health.
- Children ages two through eight need two cups of milk daily, or the equivalent in a dairy food product.
- After age nine, you need three cups of milk daily, or the equivalent.
- Dairy foods bolster bone health and help fight high blood pressure.
- Some calcium-added, nondairy foods make suitable dairy substitutes.

Chapter 8

Meat and Beans

In This Chapter

- Prominent protein sources
- Safe seafood choices
- Proper portions
- Ways to limit saturated fat and cholesterol

To the untrained eye, the members of MyPyramid's Meat and Beans group are an unlikely bunch. Why is meat palling around with mixed nuts? And what do salmon and split peas have in common? There is a good reason for pairing up poultry and pistachios and for grouping tuna and tofu together. By the end of this chapter, you'll know what unites, and divides, the members of MyPyramid's Meat and Bean group. You'll also come to find out why including a variety of choices from this jam-packed group is paramount to good health.

Meet the Meat and Beans Group

It just takes a quick glance down the list of MyPyramid's Meat and Beans roster to discover that the name of the group is a bit of a misnomer. After all, the group includes poultry, fish, eggs, nuts, and seeds as well as meat and dry beans and peas. See for yourself:

Meats:

- Beef
- Bison
- Ham
- Rabbit
- Lamb
- Venison
- Pork
- Veal

Lean luncheon meats:

Lean ground meats:

- Beef
- Pork
- Lamb

Organ meats:

- Liver
- Giblets

Poultry:

- Chicken
- Duck
- Ground chicken and turkey
- Turkey
- Goose

Eggs:

- Chicken eggs
- Duck eggs

Bean burgers:

- Garden burgers
- Veggie burgers

Dry beans and peas:

- Black beans
- Falafel
- Black-eyed peas
- Kidney beans
- Chickpeas
- Lentils
- Navy beans
- Texturized vegetable protein (TVP)
- Lima beans
- Pinto beans
- Soy beans
- Split peas
- White beans
- Tofu
- Tempeh

Nuts and seeds:

- Almonds
- Peanuts
- Almond butter
- Peanut butter
- Cashews
- Pecans
- Hazelnuts (filberts)
- Pistachios
- Mixed nuts
- Pumpkin seeds
- Sesame seeds
- Sunflower seeds
- Walnuts

Fish:

Finfish such as:

- Catfish
- Pollock
- Halibut
- Snapper

- Cod
- Porgy
- Flounder
- Salmon
- Haddock
- Sea bass

- Herring
- Swordfish
- Mackerel
- Trout
- Tuna

Shellfish such as:

- Clams
- Octopus
- Crab
- Oysters
- Crayfish

- Scallops
- Lobster
- Squid (calamari)
- Mussels
- Shrimp

Canned fish such as:

- Anchovies
- Clams

- Tuna
- Sardines

Source: www.mypyramid.gov.

That is one long list. How is it possible that so many different types of foods could have one thing in common? Read on to find out.

United They Stand

You may have guessed it by now: protein is what unites meat, seafood, poultry, eggs, dry beans and peas, nuts, and seeds. Dietary protein provides calories, but energy is not its greatest asset. Protein from food supplies *amino acids*, the raw materials necessary for building bone, and for making muscle, cartilage, skin, and all other bodily substances.

Pyramid Speak

Amino acids are the building blocks of the protein in foods and bodily proteins.

Amino acids are the basis of life. When the body constructs the proteins it needs to thrive, including red and white blood cells, enzymes, and hormones, it must assemble amino acids in a specific order, with no substitutions allowed. If your body comes up short for just a single amino acid, protein construction grinds to a halt. When this happens over and over, your health suffers.

Your body produces some of the amino acids it needs to run efficiently; the remainder of the required amino acids must come from food proteins, including those found in meat, poultry, eggs, dry beans and peas, and nuts. Because the body doesn't store amino acids, you need to eat protein every day.

Beyond Protein

Protein gets top billing in the Meat and Beans group because it's what brings the group together. Protein is not the only worthy nutrient in the bunch, however. An array of foods in the Meat and Beans groups also provide a variety of nutrients.

Vitamins

The B vitamins—niacin, thiamin, riboflavin, and B6 in the foods of the Meat and Beans section—are responsible for a number of important bodily functions. They help the body release energy; play a vital role in the function of the nervous system; aid in the formation of red blood cells; and assist in building body tissues.

Vitamin E, found in nuts and seeds, is an antioxidant vitamin that helps protect vitamin A and essential fatty acids from the process of oxidation. Oxidation occurs when free radicals attack cells and cause harm. Free radicals, the by-products of normal metabolism, also form in your body in response to environmental influences, including strong ultraviolet light from the sun and air pollution.

Mighty Minerals

Iron, prevalent in animal foods, is used to ferry oxygen to your cells. Meat, poultry, clams, and oysters are among the richest food sources of heme iron, the type of iron your body absorbs the best. Heme iron is found only in animal foods.

Plant foods, including lentils, contain only non-heme iron. Non-heme iron is also the form of iron added to processed grains including infant cereals, breads, breakfast cereals, and rice. Combining a source of vitamin C, such as strawberries or orange juice, with foods containing non-heme iron improves iron absorption from food.

Fun FAQs

If you're always tired, could your diet be to blame? You may have an iron deficiency. In fact, iron deficiency anemia is the most common nutritional deficiency in America, affecting older infants, young children, and women in their childbearing years. Coming up short on iron may also curb your powers of concentration.

Like iron, animal foods, including pork, poultry, and lamb, harbor higher levels of absorbable zinc. Zinc is one busy mineral, helping to produce DNA; assisting in breaking down carbohydrate, fat, and protein for energy; acting as a part of insulin, the hormone that regulates blood glucose levels; and boosting immunity and wound healing.

The magnesium in halibut, pollock, pumpkin and sunflower seeds, cashews, lentils, and almonds rarely receives the respect it deserves. Magnesium is instrumental in building bones. It's also necessary for maintaining a normal heart beat; keeping blood pressure in check; and releasing energy from muscle tissue.

Focus on Fiber

Dry beans and peas—including navy beans, lentils, black beans, and kidney beans—are among the top fiber foods in the Meat and Beans group, and in general. The beauty of beans is that you get carbohydrate, fiber, protein, vitamins, and minerals all rolled into one food.

Searching for Saturated Fat

And now, the bad news. There is a downside to the Meat and Beans crew. Certain members pack high levels of total fat, saturated fat, and cholesterol. You must have guessed that bacon, bologna, and hot dogs weren't going to pass muster. You are no idiot.

High levels of saturated fat from food may increase your blood levels of total *low-density lipoprotein (LDL) cholesterol*, also known as "bad" cholesterol. High levels of LDL cholesterol in the bloodstream boost the risk of heart disease and stroke by contributing to clogged arteries.

Pyramid Speak

Low-density lipoprotein cholesterol languishes in arteries, initiating a process that may ultimately block the flow of oxygen-rich blood to your heart or brain.

These foods are among those rich in saturated fat:

- Fatty cuts of beef, pork, and lamb
- Regular (75% to 85% lean) ground beef
- Ground turkey and chicken (unless 100% white meat)
- Regular sausages, hot dogs, and bacon
- Luncheon meats, including regular bologna and salami
- Duck

Foods that contain saturated fat typically contain cholesterol, too, although cholesterol is found only in animal foods. Diets rich in cholesterol may raise LDL cholesterol levels in the blood, but dietary cholesterol is not nearly as capable of increasing LDL cholesterol levels as saturated fat. Certain foods in the Meat and Beans group are higher in cholesterol than others. Learn more about saturated fat and the cholesterol content of foods in Chapter 9.

Portion Sizes

You know what to eat——a variety of foods from the Meat and Beans group. The question is, how much of each can you have? Remember the ounce-equivalent idea introduced in Chapter 4? It's back! When your MyPyramid eating plan suggests how much to eat every day from the Meat and Beans group, it will be in ounce-equivalents, the amount of food equal to one ounce of meat, poultry, or seafood.

The following chart lists specific amounts that count as one-ounce equivalents in the Meat and Beans group to help you plan meals and snacks.

Food	Amount equal to one ounce-equivalent
Lean cooked beef, lean cooked pork or ham	1 ounce
Cooked chicken or turkey, no skin or bones	1 ounce
Sliced sandwich turkey meat	1 slice

Food	Amount equal to one ounce-equivalent
Cooked fish or shellfish	1 ounce
Eggs	1 whole
Nuts	½ ounce: 12 almonds or 24 pistachios or 7 walnut halves
Seeds	½ ounce
Almond butter	1 tablespoon
Peanut butter	1 tablespoon
Cooked dry beans	¼ cup
Cooked dry peas	¼ cup
Baked beans, refried beans	¼ cup
Lentil soup	½ cup
Split pea soup	½ cup
Bean soup	½ cup
Tofu	¼ cup (about 2 ounces)
Tempeh, cooked	1 ounce
Roasted soybeans	¼ cup
Falafel patty	1 (about 4 ounces)
Hummus	2 tablespoons

Source: www.mypyramid.gov.

There are dozens of ways to use the foods from the Meat and Beans group to make meals and snacks more interesting and varied. Read on to learn more about breaking out of your food rut.

Mix It Up!

Many people do not make a variety of choices from the Meat and Beans group. They'd rather stick to grilled boneless skinless chicken breast for dinner every night, because it's easy to prepare and they think chicken is good for them to eat nearly every day. Some people eschew health concerns, and pile on the fatty meats at nearly every meal.

There's really no excuse to eat either way, especially now that you know what the members of the Meat and Beans group have to offer. If you still need convincing to try an array of tastes and textures, this section will help you get beyond eating just meat and poultry.

Go Nuts!

You probably love nuts, but you won't touch them for the fat and calories. And you never considered eating them in place of meat. You can now. MyPyramid gives you permission to have nuts and seeds on a daily basis. What? You heard right. There are a number of reasons why nuts and seeds should be a consistent part of your diet.

The likes of almonds, walnuts, and sunflower seeds supply polyunsaturated and monounsaturated fat. According to MyPyramid, when you eat fat, most of it should be in the unsaturated form to promote heart health. Plus, certain unsaturated fats from food are absolutely essential in the diet because your body cannot produce them on its own.

There's more to nuts and seeds than heart-healthy essential fats. Sunflower seeds, almonds, and hazelnuts (filberts) are the richest sources of vitamin E going in the Meat and Beans food group. To help meet daily vitamin E recommendations, health experts recommend eating nuts and seeds regularly, as long as you stick to the suggested amounts, that is.

 Power Point

Just 24 whole almonds (one ounce) supply about half of the vitamin E an adult needs every day.

Is an Egg a Day Okay?

If you've been avoiding eggs because of their cholesterol content, you can stop now. You may actually be doing yourself a disservice by keeping eggs off your plate.

Scientific evidence suggests most people can consume a whole egg—yes, yolk included——every day without raising their risk of heart disease. That's good news because the bulk of an egg's nutrition is located in the yolk. Eggs provide an array of vitamins and minerals, never mind their stellar protein content. Eggs have the highest-quality protein of any food; egg protein is used as the standard for comparing all other food proteins for their ability to promote growth and sustain life.

Eggs have something most other members of the Meat and Beans group do not: choline. Choline is not a vitamin or a mineral and it doesn't provide any calories. So what does it do for you? Choline plays a key role in memory function in fetal brain development and may head off certain birth defects during pregnancy.

Eggs are the second best source of choline, surpassed only by beef liver. One large egg satisfies about half an adult's daily choline quota, as established by the Institute of Medicine of the National Academy of Sciences. Choline is also found in much lesser amounts in a wide variety of other foods, including cauliflower, iceberg lettuce, peanuts, and peanut butter.

A Hill of Beans

Dry beans and peas are part of MyPyramid's Vegetables group, and they are also part of the Meat and Beans group. What gives? Beans and peas do double duty in the MyPyramid eating scheme.

Because beans and peas are packed with so much nutrition, everyone, including people who also eat meat, poultry, seafood, and eggs regularly, should include them in their eating plan on a regular basis. If you are one of those people, MyPyramid advises counting dry beans and peas as part of your vegetable allowance.

If you seldom, or never, eat the animal foods from the Meat and Beans group, see Chapter 10 for more on vegetarian diets.

Fishin' for Nutrition

Fish and seafood supply protein and several B vitamins. Plus, seafood is relatively low in calories,
cholesterol, and saturated fat. Speaking of fat, certain cold-water fish, including salmon, trout, sardines, and herring, harbor the highest amounts of a
type of polyunsaturated known as omega-3 fats.
The omega-3 fats in fish are commonly called EPA,
short for eicosapentaenoic acid, and DHA, short
for docosahexaeonoic acid.

There is scientific evidence suggesting eating fish
rich in EPA and DHA on a regular basis may
reduce the risk for dying from cardiovascular disease. The American Heart Association recommends
eating two fish meals a week for the health benefits.

Navigating Seafood Safety

Seafood, including finfish and shellfish, is healthy—
to a point. Certain fish contain contaminants that
are hazardous to your well-being, particularly if you
are a woman in your childbearing years; you're pregnant or nursing; or you are a small child.

Methyl mercury in fish, especially larger species of
fish, is a major health concern. Mercury accumu-
lates in your body. It's most problematic during
pregnancy and lactation, when mom is capable of
passing along mercury to her baby, harming his
developing nervous system.

The Food and Drug Administration (FDA) and the
Environmental Protection Agency (EPA) advise

women who may become pregnant; pregnant women; nursing mothers; and young children to avoid shark, swordfish, king mackerel, and tilefish—fish that are known to have high methyl mercury levels. Albacore or "white" tuna is not on the FDA's do-not-eat list, but the agency does suggest restricting intake to six ounces a week. Canned light tuna contains far less mercury than white.

> **Pitfalls**
>
> While younger women and small children are most vulnerable to the effects of mercury, women past their childbearing years, and men, are also prone to mercury poisoning.

What fish can you safely eat? The most vulnerable populations, previously mentioned, should be limited to 12 ounces weekly of a variety of fish with the least amount of mercury—including canned light tuna, salmon, pollock, catfish, and shrimp. Fish sticks and fast-food sandwiches are good choices because they are commonly made from fish low in mercury, including farmed catfish. That's good advice for the rest of us, too.

For more information about contaminants in fish, visit the Environmental Working Group at www.ewg.org.

Breaking Out

You're ready to broaden your eating horizons by making different choices from the Meat and Beans group. Here are some ways to make meal planning more interesting:

- Switch to grilled turkey cutlets or tenderloin as a change from chicken.

- Add canned tuna or salmon to salads.

- Try smoked salmon on a whole wheat bagel.

- Order grilled or broiled fish when dining out.

- Make chili with half the ground beef or 100% ground turkey breast, and twice the beans.

- Stir-fry vegetables and tofu.

- Snack on roasted soy nuts.

- Choose split pea, lentil, minestrone, or white bean soups more often.

- Have fat-free baked beans as a side dish.

- Feast on black-bean enchiladas.

- Toss garbanzo or kidney beans into your salad.

- Make brown rice or wild rice and beans as a main course.

- Choose veggie burgers or garden burgers instead of beef burgers.

- Snack on hummus and whole grain crackers.

- Choose nuts as a snack, on salads, or in main dishes.

- Use nuts to replace meat or poultry.

- Add slivered almonds to steamed vegetables, salads, smoothies, and breakfast cereals.

- Add toasted peanuts or cashews to a vegetable stir fry instead of meat.

- Concoct trail mix from dried fruit, roasted soy nuts, and sunflower seeds.

- Sprinkle chopped walnuts on top of low-fat ice cream or frozen yogurt.

- Add chopped walnuts or pecans to a green salad or chicken salad made with reduced-fat mayonnaise.

- Snack on pistachio nuts instead of chips.

- Keep hard-boiled eggs on hand to eat as snacks or to add to salads and sandwiches.

Keep It Lean

Many of the food choices in the Meat and Beans group, including legumes, fish, and chicken breast, are naturally low in fat. Others are not that lean. To control calories and fat, choose the leanest cuts of meat possible. Here's how.

- Go for ground beef with a label that reads 90% lean, or higher.

- Choose pork loin, tenderloin, center loin, and ham for the least amount of fat.

- Purchase skinless chicken parts, or take off the skin before cooking. Boneless skinless chicken breasts and turkey cutlets are the leanest poultry choices.

- Opt for lean turkey, roast beef, ham, or low-fat luncheon meats for sandwiches instead of fattier meats, including regular bologna or salami.

- Avoid processed meats such as ham, sausage, hot dogs, and *low-fat* luncheon or deli meats for the fat and added sodium.

- Trim away all of the visible fat from meats and poultry before cooking, and after.

- Broil, grill, roast, poach, or boil meat, poultry, or fish instead of frying.

- Drain off any fat that appears during cooking.

- Skip or limit the breading on meat, poultry, or fish. Breading adds calories. When breaded meat, poultry, or fish is fried, it soaks up fat, further increasing calorie content.

When selecting beef, look for the following terms to get the lowest-fat cuts possible:

Eye round roast, select	Short loin
Bottom round roast	Top loin strip steak, select
Round tip roast, select	Top loin strip steak, choice
Top round roast, choice	Short loin, T-bone steak, choice
Tenderloin	Top sirloin, choice
Ribeye, choice	Flank, average all grades
Arm pot roast, braised, select	
Arm pot roast, choice	

The Least You Need to Know

- Meat and Beans as a food group includes meat, poultry, seafood, dry beans and peas, eggs, nuts, and seeds.
- Protein is common to all foods found in the Meat and Beans category.
- Choose lean meat and poultry more often than fattier cuts.
- Opt for a wide selection of seafood, beans, nuts, seeds, and eggs instead of eating just meat and poultry at meals.

◆ Women in their childbearing years and small children must avoid shark, swordfish, king mackerel, and tilefish because of high mercury levels.

Chapter 9

Fats and Oils

In This Chapter

- Discover different types of fat
- Learn how fat and cholesterol influence health
- Distinguish between oils and solid fats
- Find out oil serving sizes

Face it: Fat makes food taste good. Really good. The olive oil in Italian food, the butter in cookies, and the peanut oil that seasons stir-fried meat and vegetable dishes is what makes food worth eating. Fat also adds to eating satisfaction by keeping you fuller longer.

You may think of fat as the forbidden nutrient. It's not. Yes, fat is linked to certain chronic conditions that plague Americans, including obesity. Yet some kinds of fat actually contribute to good health. Confused? This chapter sorts out the good fat from the bad, fills you in on MyPyramid's fat portion sizes, and helps you trim fat without sacrificing taste.

Fat Facts

There are three different types of fat found in the foods you eat: saturated, polyunsaturated, and monounsaturated. A fourth type, called trans fat, is largely produced during food processing, although trace amounts can be found naturally in full-fat dairy foods and fatty meats.

All fats supply nine calories per gram. That's more than twice the calories of carbohydrate or protein, the other energy-providing nutrients in foods. Different types of fat affect your health in different ways. Put simply, there are good fats and bad fats.

Good: Unsaturated Fats

Unsaturated fats supply essential fatty acids. You learned that in Chapter 8. As part of a balanced diet, polyunsaturated fats are also beneficial because they help keep blood cholesterol levels within a normal range. Normal blood cholesterol concentrations contribute to clear arteries that help head off heart disease and stroke.

Polyunsaturated fats are found in foods such as soybean, corn, safflower, and sunflower oil. They are also prevalent in seafood as omega-3 fats. Like polyunsaturated fat, monounsaturated fat is considered heart-healthy. Monounsaturated fat is found in canola, olive, and peanut oils, as well as in avocado, nuts, and nut butters.

Bad: Saturated Fat

Animal and plant foods supply saturated fat in varying levels, although high-fat meats and dairy foods are the worst offenders. Coconut, palm, palm kernel oil, and cocoa butter—used in processed foods including cookies, crackers, and candy—also pack saturated fat.

You make all the saturated fat your body needs, so you don't require saturated fat from food. That's not to say saturated fat is forbidden. But problems arise when people consume too much saturated fat from foods, putting them at risk for *atherosclerosis*, a condition that leads to heart attack and stroke in most, but not all, people.

 Pyramid Speak

Atherosclerosis contributes to clogged arteries by encouraging deposits of fatty substances, cholesterol, and other junk in arteries to the point of narrowing them significantly or completely blocking them. Blocked arteries reduce the flow of oxygen-rich blood to the heart and brain.

Bad: Trans Fat

Trans fat, found primarily in processed foods such as margarine, shortening, donuts and other pastries, microwave popcorn, cookies, french fries, crackers, and granola bars is the result of an industrial process. Although fatty meats and full-fat dairy foods contain some trans fats, it's clear that processed foods provide the lion's share of trans fat in the American diet.

You don't need trans fat. In fact, trans fats may be even worse for your health than the saturated fat in foods. Trans fats block the clearance of cholesterol from your bloodstream, contributing to a build up that clogs arteries and leads to stroke and heart disease. Health experts suggest eating as little trans fat as possible. Look for trans fat content on Nutrition Facts panels on processed foods.

> **Fun FAQs**
>
> What transforms fat into trans fat? Hydrogenation, which forces hydrogen into vegetable oils, transforming unsaturated fats into trans fats. Hydrogenation creates tastier, firmer fats with a longer shelf life, which is considered ideal for processed foods.

Oils

When MyPyramid specifies added fat, it means oils. There's a good reason for that. Oils from plant sources are cholesterol-free and they typically pack polyunsaturated and monounsaturated fat. In addition to the essential fatty acids they contain, oils are the major source of vitamin E in our diet.

It doesn't take a genius to figure out that oils are fats in liquid form, or pourable at room temperature, such as canola oil and olive oil. Seems straightforward, right? Sure. But this next part is a little trickier and may be harder to grasp.

Mayonnaise, salad dressing, and soft (tub) margarine with no trans fat do not fit the pourable profile, yet they are included in MyPyramid's oil allowance. Just to confuse matters, nuts, seeds, olives, and avocados are included, too. Why? They contain oil.

Moving on to the next fat fact you must know, coconut oil and palm kernel oil are not included in MyPyramid's oils category, despite fitting the pourable-at-room-temperature criteria. Here's why. These "tropical oils" are so high in saturated fat that MyPyramid regards them as solid fats because of their potential health effects.

 Power Point

Butter or stick margarine? MyPyramid says: neither is the best choice. Go for tub margarine that's free of trans fat.

Solid Fats

Solid fats are fats that are solid at room temperature, including butter and shortening, and the visible fat on meat. Solid fats come naturally from a number of animal foods. Vegetable oils can be transformed into solid fats by hydrogenation. Some common solid fats are:

- ◆ Butter
- ◆ Beef fat (tallow, suet)
- ◆ Chicken fat

- ◆ Pork fat (lard)
- ◆ Stick margarine
- ◆ Shortening

Pyramid Speak

Solid fats are solid at room temperature, such as butter, lard, and shortening, and contain high levels of saturated fat. Certain oils, including coconut oil and palm kernel oil, are lumped in with solid fats because of their saturated fat content.

Solid fats may contain cholesterol and are higher in saturated fat than most oils. In some cases, the solid fat in food is invisible. Most of the time, foods with invisible solid fats are rich in total fat, saturated fat, and cholesterol. Here are some examples:

- ◆ Full-fat cheese
- ◆ Cream
- ◆ Ice cream
- ◆ Fatty cuts of beef
- ◆ Baked goods (cookies, crackers, donuts, pastries, and croissants)

- ◆ Regular ground beef
- ◆ Bacon
- ◆ Sausages
- ◆ Poultry skin

Fat Portions

Granted, some oils are good for you. There is a point of diminishing returns, however. Too much healthy oil can contribute to weight gain that could lead to ill health.

You may use up your oils allowance in a variety of ways. It's easier to measure the oil you eat when it's plain, such as the olive oil you use in cooking or as salad dressing. This chart makes it easier to figure your oil use when it comes to fatty foods, such as margarine and mayonnaise.

Food	Amount	Amount of oil
Oils:		
Vegetable oils	1 tablespoon	3 teaspoons
Foods rich in oils:		
Margarine, soft (trans free)	1 tablespoon	2½ teaspoons
Mayonnaise	1 tablespoon	2½ teaspoons
Mayonnaise-type salad dressing	1 tablespoon	1 teaspoon
Italian dressing	2 tablespoons	2 teaspoons
Thousand Island dressing	2 tablespoons	2½ teaspoons
Olives, ripe, canned	4 large	½ teaspoon
Avocado	½ medium	3 teaspoons
Peanut butter	2 tablespoons	4 teaspoons

continues

continued

Food	Amount	Amount of oil
Peanuts, dry roasted	1 ounce	3 teaspoons
Cashews, dry roasted	1 ounce	3 teaspoons
Almonds, dry roasted	1 ounce	3 teaspoons
Hazelnuts	1 ounce	4 teaspoons
Sunflower seeds	1 ounce	3 teaspoons

Source: www.mypyramid.gov.

Oils pack lots of calories into a small space. That's why you need to temper your love of fatty foods with your need to achieve and maintain a healthy weight. You don't have to give up fatty foods entirely, however, especially if they supply healthy fats.

Striking a Fat Balance

Most of us have a preference for fatty foods, so we have no trouble working in the fat we need. That's one of the reasons Americans are facing an obesity epidemic. Fat is a concentrated source of energy that goes down easily as a hidden part of foods or as part of a topping for foods, including dressings and sauces.

That does not mean a very low-fat diet is the answer for good health. Inadequate fat intake may mean a deficiency of essential fatty acids, resulting in scaly skin and other problems. Shortchanging a child of essential fatty acids may lead to poor

growth and development, because it robs them of
the calories they need, as well as visual and neuro-
logical abnormalities.

Here's how to start weaning yourself off some of
your favorite high-fat foods.

Swap this	For this
Oil for sautéing	Broth
Coffee smoothie drink	Iced latte with fat-free milk
Full-fat milk	1% low-fat or fat-free milk
Hamburger	100% ground turkey breast burger
French fries	Mashed potatoes with low-fat milk
Chocolate chip cookies	Fig bars and graham crackers
Muffin or doughnut	Whole grain bagel
Premium ice cream	Low-fat frozen yogurt
Bacon	Canadian bacon
Stuffed-crust cheese pizza	Thin-crust cheese pizza topped with meat

Consider Cholesterol

Cholesterol is not a type of fat. It doesn't even provide any energy in the form of calories. Yet without
it, life would be impossible.

Cholesterol is part of every cell; it's the building
block for hormones, including estrogen (the primary

female sex hormone) and testosterone (the primary male hormone); the bile acids that aid digestion, and vitamin D, critical for calcium absorption and bone strength. Cholesterol is also part of myelin, the sheath that surrounds and protects your nerve cells. You make all the cholesterol your body requires, so you don't actually need to eat any. Unless you're a strict vegetarian, it's next to impossible to avoid eating cholesterol.

Too much cholesterol is blamed for blocking arteries that lead to the heart and brain. But that belies the much stronger effect of saturated fat on your risk of heart attack and stroke. Saturated fat is by far the greater culprit in hiking blood cholesterol concentrations. Cholesterol is often guilty by association because it is found in the same foods that pack excessive amounts of saturated fat, including fatty meats and dairy foods.

Health experts recommend limiting dietary cholesterol to 300 milligrams on average every day, although it's unclear exactly why this level is considered beneficial. The following chart will help you compute cholesterol intake.

Food	Portion	Cholesterol (milligrams)
Beef liver	3 oz.	324
Whole egg, medium	1	186
Egg white, medium	1	0
Fast-food chili	1 c.	170
Beef, bottom round, cooked	3 oz.	84

Food	Portion	Cholesterol (milligrams)
Danish pastry (fruit)	1	81
Soft-serve ice cream, vanilla	½ c.	81
Pork chop	3 oz.	78
Ground beef, 80% lean, cooked	3 oz.	77
Chicken breast, skinless, cooked	3 oz.	73
Turkey breast, skinless, cooked	3 oz.	72
Haddock, cooked	3 oz.	66
Salmon, cooked	3 oz.	60
Whole milk ricotta cheese	½ c.	63
Part-skim ricotta cheese	½ c.	38
Scallops, cooked	3 oz.	45
Yogurt, whole milk, plain	1 c.	32
Yogurt, low-fat, plain	1 c.	15
Yogurt, fat-free, plain	1 c.	5
Butter	1 T.	31
Cheddar cheese	1 oz.	30
Whole milk	1 c.	24
2% reduced-fat milk	1 c.	20
1% reduced-fat milk	1 c.	10
Fat-free milk	1 c.	4
Cream cheese	1 T.	16
Mayonnaise, regular	1 T.	4
Mayonnaise, low-fat	1 T.	4

Cholesterol is found only in animal foods. As you can see from the chart, lower-fat foods generally supply less cholesterol.

The Least You Need to Know

- Oils are MyPyramid's preferred added fat source.
- Oils are richer in unsaturated fats than solid fats.
- Unsaturated fats are healthier than saturated or trans fats.
- You need some unsaturated fat to survive.
- Your body does not require saturated or trans fats; both are considered unhealthy.
- You make all the cholesterol your body needs, so you don't require any from the foods you eat.

Chapter 10

Eating on the Run

In This Chapter

- ◆ Find nutritious foods to take with you
- ◆ Identify healthy portion sizes
- ◆ Cut calories when dining out
- ◆ Figure mixed dishes into a MyPyramid eating plan

If you're like most people, you "dine" away from home more than ever, whether it's downing an airport meal before catching a plane; chowing breakfast, lunch, or dinner while driving in the car; or snacking at malls or the museum.

You're always eating on the run, so you couldn't possibly eat a balanced diet, right? Not so fast. Even with your hectic schedule, it's possible to hold on to your resolve to eat better by following one of the 12 MyPyramid eating plans. You just need a few simple strategies for eating on the run. This chapter spells them out for you.

Practice Portion Control

Restaurant fare will nearly always dish up more calories, fat, and sodium than what you make at home. And don't forget about the larger-than-you-should-eat portions. When it comes to weight control, servings matter. The good news is that you can eat any type of food when you're dining out. As long as you don't overindulge, you'll probably be successful at weight control.

Chances are, you won't be lugging your food scale, measuring cups, and spoons on a business trip, vacation, or trip to the mall. So this handy chart will help you estimate serving sizes when you can't measure your food.

This amount of food	Looks like
3 ounces meat, poultry, or fish	A deck of playing cards
½ cup of fruit, vegetables, pasta, rice, or breakfast cereal	The amount that fits into a small fist
1 ice cream serving	The amount that would fit into your open hand
1 ounce of cheese; 1 tablespoon of butter, oil, salad dressing, or margarine	The size of your thumb
1 teaspoon of margarine, butter, oil, or salad dressing	The tip of your thumb to the first knuckle

Of course, eating small portions of whatever you want doesn't guarantee a balanced diet. Restaurant meals are typically lower in fruits, vegetables, and whole grains. That really doesn't matter much if you dine out occasionally, but if you're eating away from home often, restaurant fare can easily take a toll on your health.

Make a Plan

If you feel like you're always eating on the fly, you probably are. You need a game plan, complete with coping strategies. When you're out and about more often than not, pack some healthy foods, using MyPyramid portion sizes as your guide, to have on hand in your briefcase or in the car. Following are some suggestions for foods that don't need refrigeration.

- Dried fruit
- Nuts
- Light popcorn
- Whole grain crackers

- Whole fresh fruit
- Tomato juice in cans (6 oz.)
- Peanut butter in a tube

Take these along in a small cooler or refrigerated bag:

- Yogurt, in a tube or cup
- Cheese sticks
- Cut fruit

- Sandwiches
- Orange juice

Order Up!

Most of us eat the same types of foods in the same types of restaurants. In a way, that makes it easier for you to eat right, unless you favor fried-clam shacks and rib joints. Identify restaurants that have lighter, healthier fare, including grilled chicken and seafood, and stick with them. Then use these tips to work in even more nutrition when dining out.

- Instead of regular soda, order water or fat-free or low-fat milk, unsweetened tea, or other drinks without added sugars.
- Split an entrée with a friend.
- Order two low-fat appetizers or a low-fat appetizer and a salad for dinner instead of a larger entrée.
- Request whole grain bread or bagels for sandwiches or toast.
- Start your meal with a garden salad packed with veggies to curb your appetite and work in some produce.
- Take one piece of bread or a roll and have the bread basket removed from your table so you don't overdo it.
- Ask for salad dressing to be served on the side so that you can control the serving size.
- Opt for entrées that include vegetables, such as stir-fries, kabobs, or pasta with a tomato sauce.
- Ask for a doggy bag as soon as your food arrives at the table to prevent picking at the large portions left over on your plate.
- Order steamed, grilled, or broiled dishes instead of those that are fried or sautéd.
- Skip all-you-can-eat buffets. They encourage overeating.
- Avoid foods with creamy sauces or gravies.
- Avoid adding oil or butter to your foods.
- Choose a fruit-based dessert.
- Split high-calorie desserts with a friend, or three.

Fun FAQs

Is it okay to bank some calories to save for a restaurant meal? Yes. Skim a few hundred discretionary calories the day before, the day of, and the day after your big night out. Add more exercise to help keep you on track.

What's on the Menu?

Dining out is your passion. How do you eat away from home following a balanced diet? It's not easy, especially when restaurant food is full of pitfalls. You'll do a better job of avoiding calories with some ordering savvy. Here's how:

Type: Chinese Food

Drawbacks: Copious quantities of oil in stir-fry dishes and deep-fried fare. High-fat meats, including spare ribs and fried chicken and shrimp.

You should: Order plain rice instead of fried rice and high-fat noodle dishes. Use chopsticks to eat more slowly. Opt for stir-fry poultry or seafood and vegetable dishes.

Type: Italian Food

Drawbacks: Large portions, lots of cheese, and liberal use of olive oil.

You should: Split an entrée. Order fresh vegetables as side dishes. Order plainer entrées, including pasta with marinara sauce or fresh tomato sauce, or grilled chicken or meat and vegetables.

Power Point

For information about the calories in restaurant food, visit www.calorieking.com. All of the large chain restaurants and coffee shops also have their own websites with nutrition information for their products.

Type: Fast Food

Drawbacks: Lots of fat in most of the foods. And just the smell of French fries can quickly melt your resolve to eat right.

You should: Order a grilled chicken sandwich minus the mayonnaise; a bowl of chili; fruit cup or fruit bowl with yogurt; and 100% fruit juice or low-fat milk.

Type: Mexican Food

Drawbacks: Packs fat as cheese and added oil; offers few fresh vegetables.

You should: Remove the chips from the table as soon as you sit down. Order bean soup or chili and a salad for your meal. Skip the condiments, including sour cream. Stick with cheese and bean enchiladas and pull off most of the cheese.

Type: American Food

Drawbacks: Large portions of potentially high-fat foods. (Can you say 24-ounce steak?)

You should: Split entrées. Order a side of cooked vegetables. Consider two appetizers instead of an entrée, and make one of them a large garden salad. Sip low-fat milk or 100% fruit juice.

Type: Pizza Joint

Drawbacks: Cheese, pepperoni, sausage, and any other topping that is not a vegetable.

You should: Order thin-crust cheese or vegetable pizza along with a large garden salad to help fill you up.

Considering Cocktails

Alcoholic beverages are calorie budget-busters. When you only have 2,000 calories a day to spend, there's not a lot of room for drinks with at least 150 calories, alcoholic or not. Be forewarned: you must account for the calories in beverages to stay within your MyPyramid plan calorie allowance. An occasional drink or two with a restaurant meal won't make a difference in your diet. Any more may prolong weight-loss efforts and make it more difficult and harder to keep the pounds from creeping on.

Light beer and wine are among the lowest-calorie options. To cut calories further, order a wine spritzer of half wine, half club soda. One and a half ounces of 80-proof distilled liquor, such as rum, gin, vodka, and whiskey, contains about 100 calories. The fruit juice, regular soft drinks, tonic

water, full-fat milk, and cream that you mix with
distilled spirits ups calorie content considerably.
For example, a mixed drink made from cream and
coffee brandy contains upwards of 500 calories.

Power Point _____

> You may be in the habit of ordering a
> cocktail as you sit down to a restaurant
> meal. Cut alcohol calories by starting with
> a calorie-free beverage, such as a diet
> soft drink or club soda with lemon or lime
> to start, and reserving one cocktail to have
> with your entrée.

All Mixed Up

One of the challenges of eating a healthy diet is
trying to fit your favorite dishes into its portion
parameters. Mixed dishes never go neatly. For
example, your Friday night cheese pizza cuts across
several of MyPyramid's food groups: the crust falls
into the Grains group, the tomato sauce is from the
Vegetables group, and the cheese falls into the Milk
group.

Food	Grains (oz. eq.)	Veg. (cups)	Fruit (cups)	Milk	Meat and Beans (oz. eq.)
Cheese pizza—thin crust (1 slice from medium pizza)	1	⅛	0	⅛	0
Lasagna (1 piece 3½" by 4")	2	⅛	0	1	1
Macaroni and cheese (1 cup, from packaged mix)	2	0	0	½	0
Chicken pot pie (8 oz. pie)	2½	¼	0	0	1½
Beef taco (2 tacos)	2½	¼	0	¼	2
Bean and cheese burrito (1)	2½	⅛	0	1	2
Egg roll (1)	½	⅛	0	0	½
Chicken fried rice (1 cup)	1½	¼	0	0	1
Stuffed peppers with rice and meat (½ pepper)	½	½	0	0	1
Beef stir-fry (1 cup)	0	¾	0	0	1
New England style clam chowder (1 cup)	½	⅛	0	½	2

continues

continued

Food	Grains (oz. eq.)	Veg. (cups)	Fruit (cups)	Milk	Meat and Beans (oz. eq.)
Manhattan style clam chowder (1 cup)	0	⅜	0	0	2
Cream of tomato soup (1 cup)	½	½	0	½	0
Large cheeseburger	2	0	0	⅓	3
Turkey sub (6" sub)	2	½	0	¼	2
Peanut butter and jelly sandwich	2	0	0	0	2
Tuna salad sandwich	2	¼	0	0	2
Chef salad (3 cups—no dressing)	0	1½	0	0	3
Pasta salad with vegetables (1 cup)	1½	½	0	0	0
Apple pie (1 slice)	2	0	¼	0	0
Pumpkin pie (1 slice)	1½	⅛	0	¼	¼

Source: www.mypyramid.gov.

The Least You Need to Know

- It is possible to eat healthy while eating on the run.

- Restaurant food contains more calories, fat, and sodium than homemade foods.

- Portion control is central to healthy dining out.

- You must account for calories consumed as beverages.

MyPyramid Plans

In This Chapter

- Choose a MyPyramid eating plan
- Discover the number of servings to eat from each food group every day
- Find sample menus for MyPyramid plans

You've read the book. Now you're ready for action. This chapter is where it all comes together. Your newfound nutrition knowledge meets up with specific recommendations for what and how much to eat every day. Your food pyramid awaits.

How to Use This Chapter

Go directly to the plan you have chosen for yourself after reading Chapters 2 and 3. Take a look at the number of servings from each food group and study the sample menu. You do not need to follow the sample menu to the letter. It's just one way to put together a balanced diet. However, when constructing a healthy diet from a MyPyramid blueprint, be sure to eat at least three meals a day.

Eating on a regular schedule helps keep you on track to make healthier food choices by preventing excessive hunger. You'll find a discretionary calorie allowance for the entire day at the end of each sample menu. See Chapter 3 for more on discretionary calories.

Write down what you eat to ensure you're getting what you need and help prevent you from eating too many high-calorie foods. Consult the Vegetable Recommendations sheet, located in Appendix C, for the details about including the suggested servings from the vegetable subgroups each week.

Eating right is a process, not an overnight miracle. Try not to feel discouraged when you don't work in all the produce or dairy foods you need, or if you indulge in too many chocolate chip cookies on occasion. Working at healthy eating is what matters most.

MyPyramid 1,000 Calories

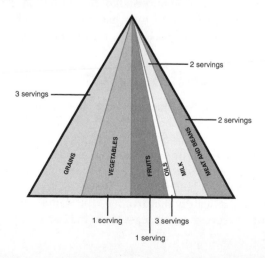

Sample Menu

Breakfast

¼ cup cooked oatmeal

1 tsp. tub margarine

½ cup low-fat milk

½ medium banana

Snack

4 ounces low-fat fruited yogurt

½ medium banana

Lunch

1 ounce cooked, skinless, boneless chicken

½ cup cooked broccoli with 1 tsp. tub margarine

1 slice whole grain bread

½ cup low-fat milk

Snack

1 ounce hard cheese

7 soda crackers

Dinner

1 ounce cooked lean beef

¼ cup cooked rice with 1 tsp. tub margarine

½ cup cooked carrots

½ cup low-fat milk

Discretionary calories: 165

My Pyramid 1,200 Calories

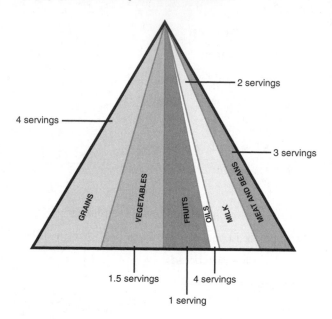

Sample Menu

Breakfast

½ cup cooked oatmeal

1 tsp. tub margarine

½ cup low-fat milk

½ medium banana

Snack

4 ounces low-fat fruited yogurt

½ medium banana

Lunch

1 ounce cooked, skinless, boneless chicken

¾ cup cooked broccoli with 1 tsp. tub margarine

2 slices whole grain bread

½ cup low-fat milk

Snack

1 ounce hard cheese

7 soda crackers

Dinner

2 ounces cooked lean beef

¼ cup cooked rice with 1 tsp. tub margarine

¾ cup cooked carrots with 1 tsp. tub margarine

½ cup low-fat milk

Discretionary calories: 171

MyPyramid 1,400 Calories

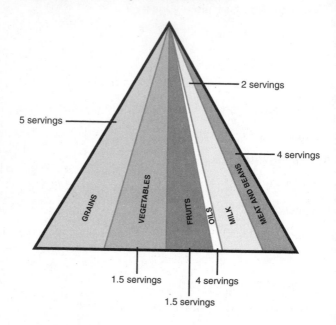

Sample Menu

Breakfast

½ cup cooked oatmeal

1 tsp. tub margarine

½ cup low-fat milk

½ medium banana

Snack

4 ounces low-fat fruited yogurt

½ medium banana

Lunch

2 ounces cooked, skinless, boneless chicken

¾ cup cooked broccoli with 1 tsp. tub margarine

2 slices whole grain bread

1 medium apple

½ cup low-fat milk

Snack

1 ounce hard cheese

7 soda crackers

Dinner

2 ounces cooked lean beef

½ cup cooked rice with 1 tsp. tub margarine

¾ cup cooked carrots with 1 tsp. tub margarine

½ cup low-fat milk

Discretionary calories: 171

MyPyramid 1,600 Calories

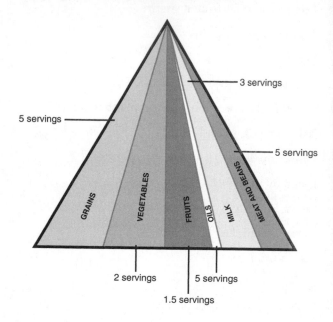

Sample Menu

Breakfast

½ cup cooked oatmeal

1 tsp. tub margarine

½ cup low-fat milk

½ medium banana

Snack

4 ounces low-fat fruited yogurt

½ medium banana

Lunch

2 ounces cooked, skinless, boneless chicken

¾ cup cooked broccoli with 2 tsp. tub margarine

2 slices whole grain bread

1 medium apple

1 cup low-fat milk

Snack

1 ounce hard cheese

7 soda crackers

12 baby carrots

Dinner

3 ounces cooked lean beef

½ cup cooked rice with 1 tsp. tub margarine

¾ cup cooked carrots with 1 tsp. tub margarine

1 cup low-fat milk

Discretionary calories: 132

MyPyramid 1,800 Calories

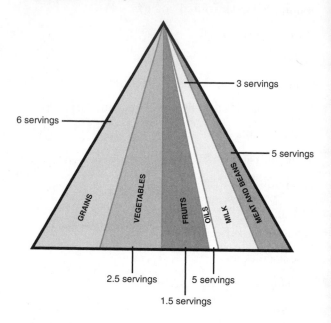

Sample Menu

Breakfast

½ cup cooked oatmeal

1 tsp. tub margarine

½ cup low-fat milk

½ medium banana

Snack

4 ounces low-fat fruited yogurt

½ medium banana

Lunch

2 ounces cooked, skinless, boneless chicken

¾ cup cooked broccoli with 2 tsp. tub margarine

2 slices whole grain bread

1 medium apple

1 cup low-fat milk

Snack

1 ounce hard cheese

7 soda crackers

12 baby carrots

Dinner

3 ounces cooked lean beef

½ cup cooked rice with 1 tsp. tub margarine

1 cup cooked carrots with 1 tsp. tub margarine

1 cup low-fat milk

Snack

3 cups low-fat popcorn, popped

Discretionary calories: 195

MyPyramid 2,000 Calories

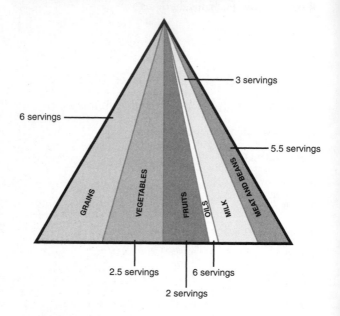

Sample Menu

Breakfast

1 cup cooked oatmeal

1 tsp. tub margarine

1 cup low-fat milk

¼ cup dried fruit

Snack

8 ounces fruited low-fat yogurt

Lunch

Salad: 2 ounces cooked, skinless, boneless chicken; 2 cups dark green leafy vegetables; ½ cup beans, such as garbanzo; ½ cup chopped tomato topped with 3 teaspoons olive oil, and balsamic vinegar

2 ounces whole grain bread

1 medium apple

Snack

1 ½ ounces hard cheese

12 baby carrots

Dinner

3½ ounces cooked lean beef

½ cup cooked rice with 1 tsp. tub margarine

1 cup cooked carrots with 1 tsp. tub margarine

Snack

3 cups low-fat popcorn, popped

Discretionary calories: 267

MyPyramid 2,200 Calories

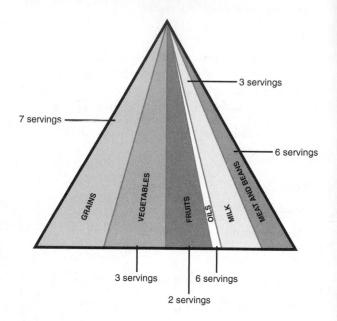

Sample Menu

Breakfast

1 cup cooked oatmeal

1 tsp. tub margarine

1 cup low-fat milk

¼ cup dried fruit

Snack

8 ounces fruited low-fat yogurt

Lunch

Salad: 2 ounces cooked, skinless, boneless chicken; 2 cups dark green leafy vegetables; ½ cup beans, such as garbanzo; ½ cup chopped tomato topped with 3 teaspoons olive oil, and balsamic vinegar

2 ounces whole grain bread

1 medium apple

Snack

1½ ounces hard cheese

12 baby carrots

7 soda crackers

Dinner

4 ounces cooked lean beef

½ cup cooked rice with 1 tsp. tub margarine

1 cup cooked carrots with 1 tsp. tub margarine

1 cup cooked broccoli

Snack

3 cups low-fat popcorn, popped

Discretionary calories: 290

MyPyramid 2,400 Calories

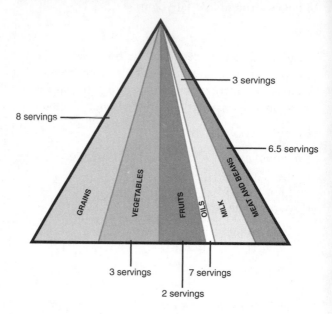

Sample Menu

Breakfast

1 cup cooked oatmeal

2 tsp. tub margarine

2 slices whole grain toast

1 cup low-fat milk

¼ cup dried fruit

Snack

8 ounces fruited low-fat yogurt

Lunch

Salad: 2½ ounces cooked, skinless, boneless chicken; 2 cups dark green leafy vegetables; ½ cup beans, such as garbanzo; ½ cup chopped tomato topped with 3 teaspoons olive oil, and balsamic vinegar

2 ounces whole grain bread

1 medium apple

Snack

1½ ounces hard cheese

12 baby carrots

7 soda crackers

Dinner

4 ounces cooked lean beef

½ cup cooked rice with 1 tsp. tub margarine

1 cup cooked carrots with 1 tsp. tub margarine

1 cup cooked broccoli

Snack

3 cups low-fat popcorn, popped

Discretionary calories: 362

MyPyramid 2,600 Calories

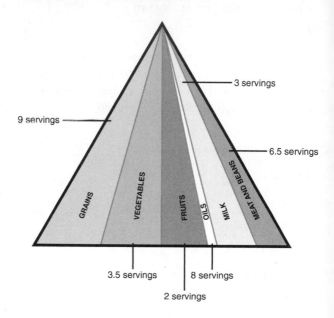

Sample Menu

Breakfast

1 cup cooked oatmeal

2 tsp. tub margarine

2 slices whole grain toast

1 cup low-fat milk

¼ cup dried fruit

Snack

8 ounces fruited low-fat yogurt

Lunch

Salad: 2½ ounces cooked, skinless, boneless chicken; 2 cups dark green leafy vegetables; ½ cup beans, such as garbanzo; ½ cup chopped tomato, and ½ cup chopped cucumber, topped with 3 teaspoons olive oil, and balsamic vinegar

2 ounces whole grain bread

1 medium apple

Snack

1½ ounces hard cheese

12 baby carrots

7 soda crackers

Dinner

4 ounces cooked lean beef

1 cup cooked rice with 1 tsp. tub margarine

1 cup cooked carrots with 1 tsp. tub margarine

1 cup cooked broccoli with 1 tsp. tub margarine

Snack

3 cups low-fat popcorn, popped

Discretionary calories: 410

MyPyramid 2,800 Calories

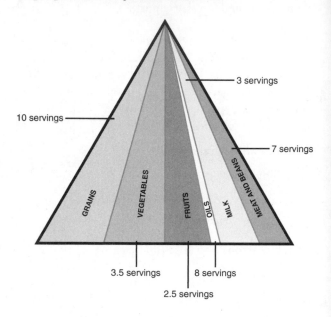

Sample Menu

Breakfast

1 cup cooked oatmeal

2 tsp. tub margarine

2 slices whole grain toast

1 hard-boiled egg

1 cup low-fat milk

¼ cup dried fruit

Snack

8 ounces fruited low-fat yogurt

½ medium banana

Lunch

Salad: 2½ ounces cooked, skinless, boneless chicken; 2 cups dark green leafy vegetables; ½ cup beans, such as garbanzo; ½ cup chopped tomato, and ½ cup chopped cucumber, topped with 3 teaspoons olive oil, and balsamic vinegar

2 ounces whole grain bread

1 medium apple

Snack

1½ ounces hard cheese

12 baby carrots

7 soda crackers

Dinner

4 ounces cooked lean beef

1 cup cooked rice with 1 tsp. tub margarine

1 cup cooked carrots with 1 tsp. tub margarine

1 cup cooked broccoli with 1 tsp. tub margarine

Snack

3 cups low-fat popcorn, popped

Discretionary calories: 426

MyPyramid 3,000 Calories

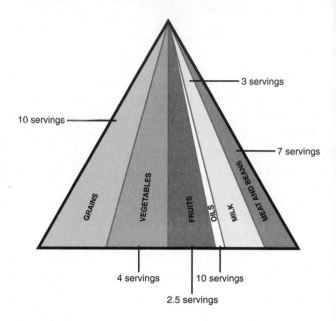

Sample Menu

Breakfast

1 cup cooked oatmeal

2 tsp. tub margarine

2 slices whole grain toast

1 hard-boiled egg

1 cup low-fat milk

¼ cup dried fruit

Snack

8 ounces fruited low-fat yogurt

½ medium banana

Lunch

Salad: 2½ ounces cooked, skinless, boneless chicken; 3 cups dark green leafy vegetables; ½ cup beans, such as garbanzo; ½ cup chopped tomato, and ½ cup chopped cucumber, topped with 4 teaspoons olive oil, and balsamic vinegar

2 ounces whole grain bread

1 medium apple with 1 tablespoon almond or peanut butter

Snack

1½ ounces hard cheese

12 baby carrots

7 soda crackers

Dinner

4 ounces cooked lean beef

1 cup cooked rice with 1 tsp. tub margarine

1 cup cooked carrots with 1 tsp. tub margarine

1 cup cooked broccoli with 1 tsp. tub margarine

Snack

3 cups low-fat popcorn, popped

Discretionary calories: 512

MyPyramid 3,200 Calories

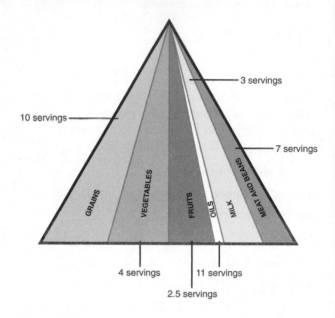

Sample Menu

Breakfast

1 cup cooked oatmeal

2 tsp. tub margarine

2 slices whole grain toast

1 hard-boiled egg

1 cup low-fat milk

¼ cup dried fruit

Snack

8 ounces fruited low-fat yogurt

½ medium banana

Lunch

Salad: 2½ ounces cooked, skinless, boneless chicken; 3 cups dark green leafy vegetables; ½ cup beans, such as garbanzo; ½ cup chopped tomato, and ½ cup chopped cucumber, topped with 4 teaspoons olive oil, and balsamic vinegar

2 ounces whole grain bread

1 medium apple with 2 tablespoons almond or peanut butter

Snack

1½ ounces hard cheese

12 baby carrots

7 soda crackers

Dinner

4 ounces cooked lean beef

1 cup cooked rice with 1 tsp. tub margarine

1 cup cooked carrots with 1 tsp. tub margarine

1 cup cooked broccoli with 1 tsp. tub margarine

Snack

3 cups low-fat popcorn, popped

Discretionary calories: 648

The Least You Need to Know

+ Stick to suggested portion sizes for calorie control.

+ Eat at least three meals a day.

+ You can design your diet in dozens of ways.

+ Choose a variety of items from within each food group.

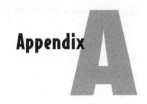

Glossary

Aerobic   Means literally "with air." Aerobic activities are repetitive and require oxygen from the air you breathe.

Allergens   Proteins found in foods not broken down during cooking or digestion that trigger the body's immune response.

Amino acids   The components of protein found in foods. Amino acids are the building blocks of body proteins, such as blood cells, muscle, and skin. Some amino acids are made by the body, while others must come from the foods you eat.

Anaerobic   Exercise that exhausts smaller muscle groups and does not require as much oxygen because the demand on the heart and lungs is not sustained.

Antioxidants   Substances including vitamins, minerals, and phytonutrients that protect cells from destructive compounds called free radicals. Antioxidants disarm free radicals, whose damage may give rise to chronic conditions including cancer and heart disease

Atherosclerosis A process that encourages deposits of fatty substances, cholesterol, and other junk in arteries to the point of narrowing them significantly or completely blocking them, leading to coronary artery disease. Blocked arteries reduce the flow of oxygen-rich blood to the heart and brain.

Body Mass Index A comparison of your height to your body weight. For most people, it's a reliable indicator of extra body fat.

Calorie A calorie is a unit of energy. The number of calories in food is determined by measuring the amount of heat it produces when burned. Your body's calorie needs are determined by gender, weight, and physical activity level.

Cholesterol A waxy, fatlike substance made by the liver and used by the body for many vital functions. Excess cholesterol in the bloodstream may contribute to coronary heart disease.

Discretionary calories The calories available to spend any way you like after you have met your nutrient needs.

Fatty acids The basic component of all types of fats. Two polyunsaturated fats, linoleic acid and linolenic acid, are considered essential fatty acids. You must get essential fatty acids from food because your body is unable to make them.

Fructose The carbohydrate in fruit and fruit juices that makes them sweet.

HDL (High-density lipoprotein cholesterol)   A type of protein-cholesterol package that helps scavenge cholesterol in the bloodstream and return it to the liver to be excreted from the body.

Homocysteine   An amino acid that's normally helpful to the body, but wreaks havoc when present in high levels. Homocysteine spells trouble for your heart and brain because it contributes to clogged arteries that block oxygen-rich blood to these vital organs.

Lactose intolerance   A condition in which your body does not make enough lactase, the enzyme necessary to break down lactose, the carbohydrate found in dairy foods.

LDL (Low-density lipoprotein cholesterol) A type of cholesterol that languishes in arteries, initiating a process that may ultimately block the flow of oxygen-rich blood to your heart or brain.

Nutrient-dense foods   Foods that provide substantial amounts of vitamins and minerals and relatively few calories.

Ounce-equivalent of grains   The amount of food considered nutritionally equal to a one-ounce slice of bread.

Ounce-equivalent of meat   The amount of food considered nutritionally equal to a one-ounce serving of meat, poultry, or seafood.

Phytonutrients   Phyto comes from the Greek word *phyton* (plant). Phytonutrients mean plant nutrients.

Refined grains Milled grains that are missing the bran and germ from the kernel along with dietary fiber, iron, and many B vitamins.

Resting metabolism The number of calories your body burns to maintain basic functions.

Solid fats Fats such as butter, lard, and shortening that are solid at room temperature and contain high levels of saturated fatty acids. Certain oils, including coconut oil and palm kernel oil, are lumped in with solid fats because of their saturated fat content.

Whole grains Grains that contain the entire grain kernel, which includes the bran, germ, and endosperm.

Resources

Books

Clark, Nancy. *Sports Nutrition Guidebook*, 3rd ed. Champaign, Illinois: Human Kinetics, 2003.

Duyff, Roberta Larsen. *The American Dietetic Association's Complete Food & Nutrition Guide*, 2nd ed. New York: John Wiley & Sons, 2002.

Fletcher, Anne M. *Thin for Life, 10 Keys to Success from People Who Have Lost Weight and Kept It Off.* New York: Houghton Mifflin, 2003.

Joseph, James A., Daniel A. Nadeau, and Anne Underwood. *The Color Code: A Revolutionary Eating Plan for Optimum Health*. New York: Hyperion, 2002.

Nelson, Miriam. *Strong Women Eat Well*. New York: Berkley Publishing Group, 2002.

O'Neil, Carolyn and Densie Webb. *The Dish on Eating Healthy and Being Fabulous!* New York: Atria Books, 2004.

Prochaska, James O., John C. Norcross, and Carlo DiClemente. *Changing for Good*. New York: Avon, 1994.

Tribole, Evelyn. *Stealth Health: How to Sneak Nutrition Painlessly into Your Diet*. New York: Penguin, 2000.

Warshaw, Hope S. *Eat Out, Eat Right!* Chicago: Surrey Books, 2003.

Newsletters

Environmental Nutrition
PO Box 420235
Palm Coast, FL 32142-0235
(800) 829-5384
www.environmentalnutrition.com

Tufts University Diet and Nutrition Letter
PO Box 57857
Boulder, CO 80322-7857
(800) 274-7581
www.healthletter.tufts.edu

Websites

Anemia www.4woman.gov/faq/anemia.htm

Coronary Heart Disease/Cardiovascular Disease www.nhlbi.nih.gov/health/public/heart/index.htm#chol

Dairy Foods www.3aday.org

Diabetes   www.fda.gov/diabetes

Dietary Guidelines for Americans, 2005
www.health.gov/dietaryguidelines/dga2005/
document/ or www.healthierus.gov/
dietaryguidelines/

Federal Government Food Safety information
www.foodsafety.gov

Food and Nutrition Information
www.nutrition.gov, www.eatright.org,
www.healthfactsandfears.com, and
www.WebMD.com

Food Composition   For data on the nutrient
content of specific foods, visit www.nal.usda.gov/
fnic/foodcomp

Food Safety Information   For information
about keeping food safe to eat, visit
www.fsis.usda.gov/Food_Safety_Education/
Food_Safety_Education_Programs/index.asp

Fruits and Vegetables   www.5aday.gov

High Blood Pressure   www.nhlbi.nih.gov/health/
public/heart/index.htm#hbp or www.nhlbi.nih.gov/
health/dci/Diseases/Hbp/HBP_WhatIs.html

Mercury in Fish   www.cfsan.fda.gov/~dms/
admehg3.html

MyPyramid   www.mypyramid.gov

Neural Tube Defects www.nlm.nih.gov/
medlineplus/neuraltubedefects.html#
preventionscreening

Nutrition Facts Label For more information
about understanding and using the Nutrition Facts
label on food products, visit www.cfsan.fda.gov/
~dms/foodlab.html

Obesity and Maintaining Healthy Weight
www.nhlbi.nih.gov/health/public/heart/index.htm#
obesity, www.nhlbi.nih.gov/health/public/
heart/obesity/lose_wt/index.htm, and www.win.
niddk.nih.gov

Osteoporosis www.fda.gov/fdac/features/
796_bone.html

Physical Activity For information about physical
activity and health, visit www.cdc.gov/nccdphp/
dnpa/physical/index.htm, www.americaonthemove.
org, www.justmove.org, and www.collagevideo.com

Vegetarian Eating www.vrg.org

Vegetable Recommendations

MyPyramid eating plans stress the importance of selecting a variety of vegetables over the course of a week. This chart shows you how to divide up your choices over a 7-day period. Look for your chosen calorie level, and then read down to find out how many servings you need from each vegetable subgroup over a week's time.

MyPyramid Calorie Level

	1,000	1,200	1,400	1,600	1,800	2,000
Dark Green	1	1.5	1.5	2	3	3
Orange	.5	1	1	1.5	2	2
Legumes	.5	1	1	2.5	3	3
Starchy	1.5	2.5	2.5	2.5	3	3
Other	3.5	4.5	4.5	5.5	6.5	6.5

	2,200	2,400	2,600	2,800	3,000	3,200
Dark Green	3	3	3	3	3	3
Orange	2	2	2.5	2.5	2.5	2.5
Legumes	3	3	3.5	3.5	3.5	3.5
Starchy	6	6	7	7	9	9
Other	7	7	8.5	8.5	10	10

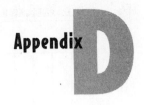

MyPyramid Worksheet

Use this worksheet to track your food intake and physical activity. Make copies of this worksheet to use on a daily basis. Research shows keeping a food journal helps with weight control, probably because seeing how much you eat means you're accountable for it. With time, writing down your food intake and physical activity may help you reach, and maintain, your goals.

Food Group	Daily Portions	Today's Choices	Daily (Goals)	Total											
Grains															
Vegetables															

Food Group	Daily Portions	Today's Choices	Daily (Goals)	Total
Fruits				
Milk				
Meat and Beans				

Food Group	Daily Portions	Today's Choices	Daily (Goals)	Total
Oils				
Extras:				
Physical Activity: Goal is at least 30 minutes each day.				
Your minutes today:				

Index

M